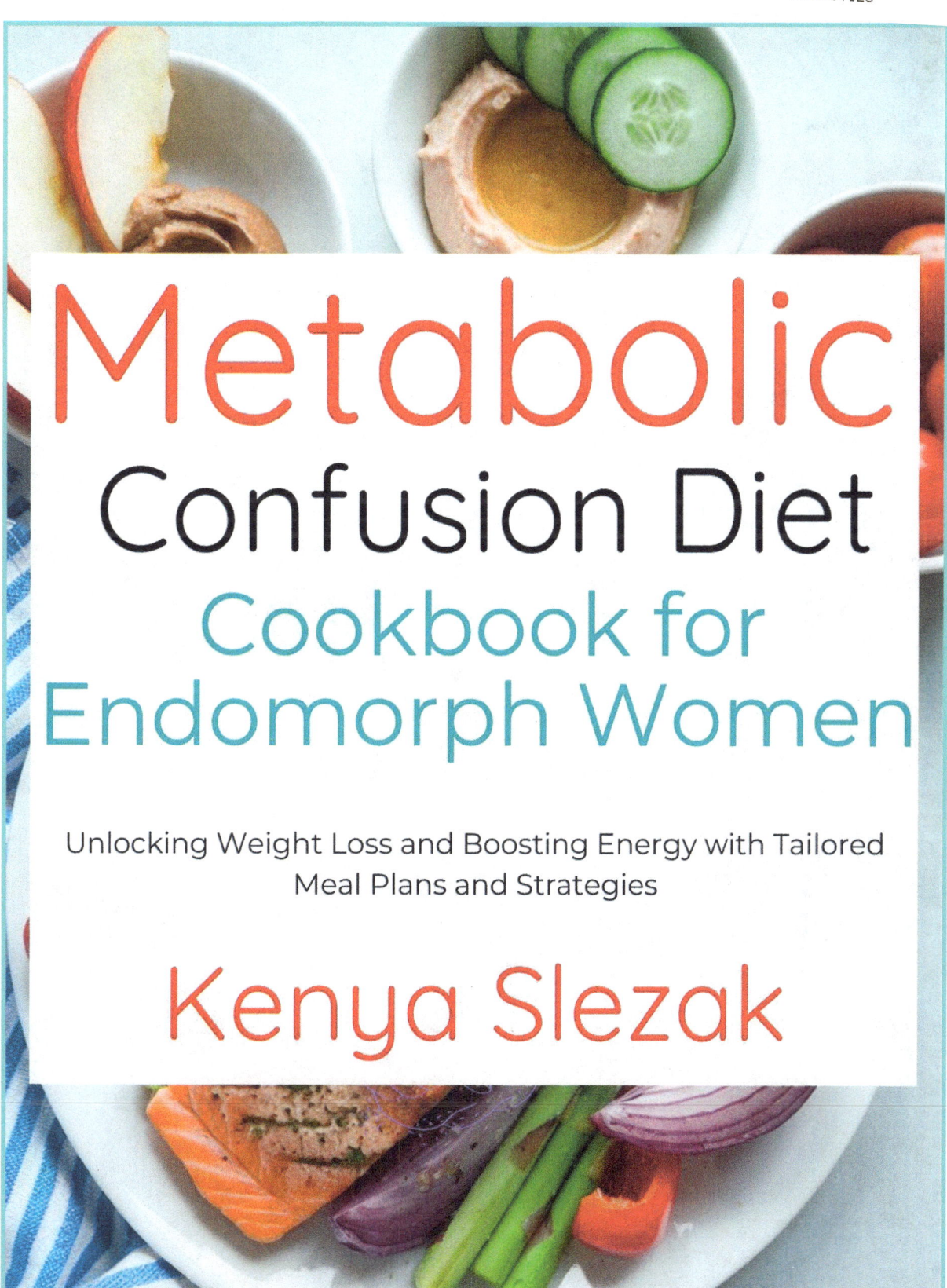

Metabolic Confusion Diet
Cookbook for Endomorph Women

Unlocking Weight Loss and Boosting Energy with Tailored Meal Plans and Strategies

Kenya Slezak

1

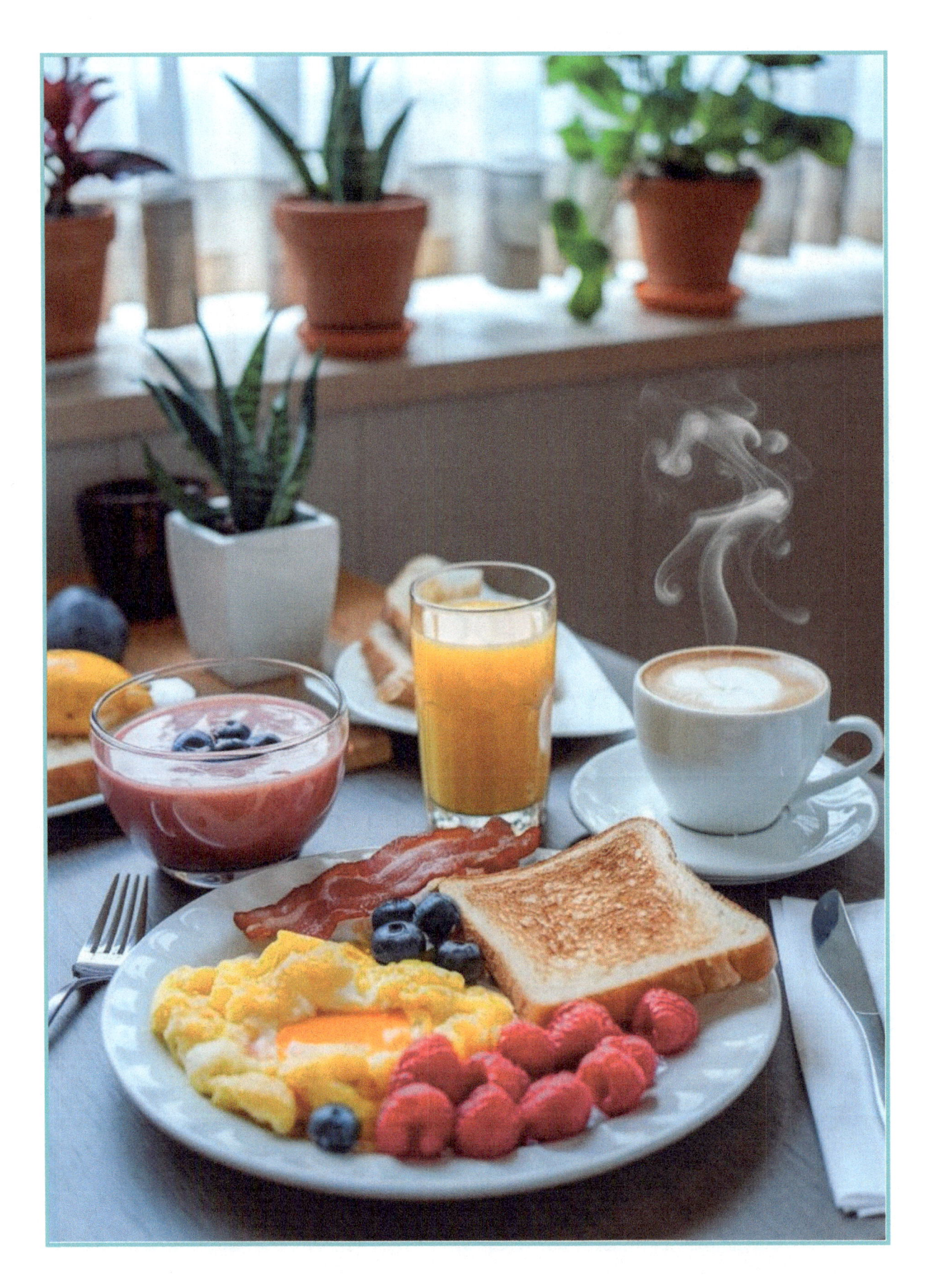

Copyright © 2025 by Kenya Slezak

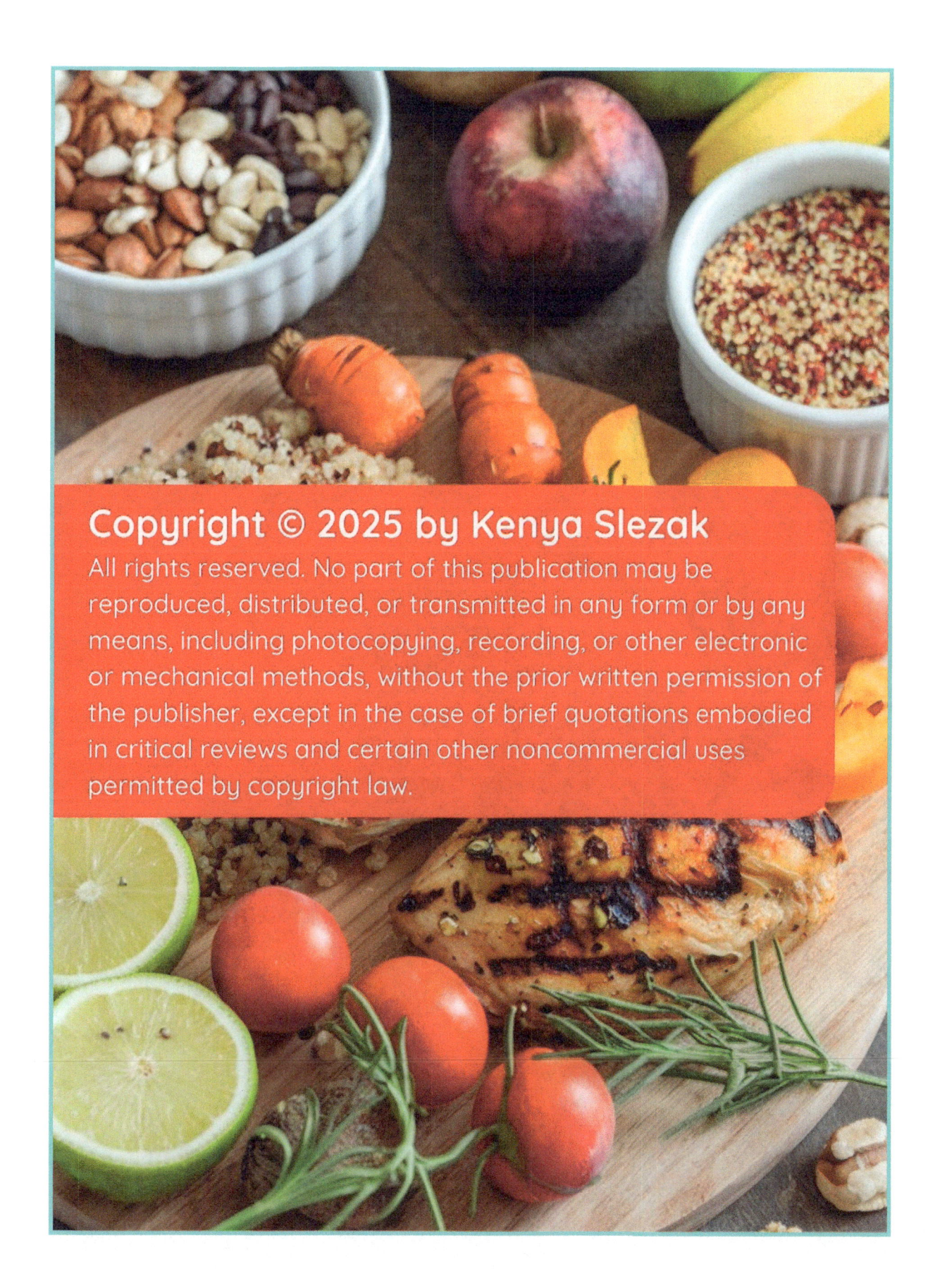

All rights reserved. No part of this publication may be reproduced, distributed, or transmitted in any form or by any means, including photocopying, recording, or other electronic or mechanical methods, without the prior written permission of the publisher, except in the case of brief quotations embodied in critical reviews and certain other noncommercial uses permitted by copyright law.

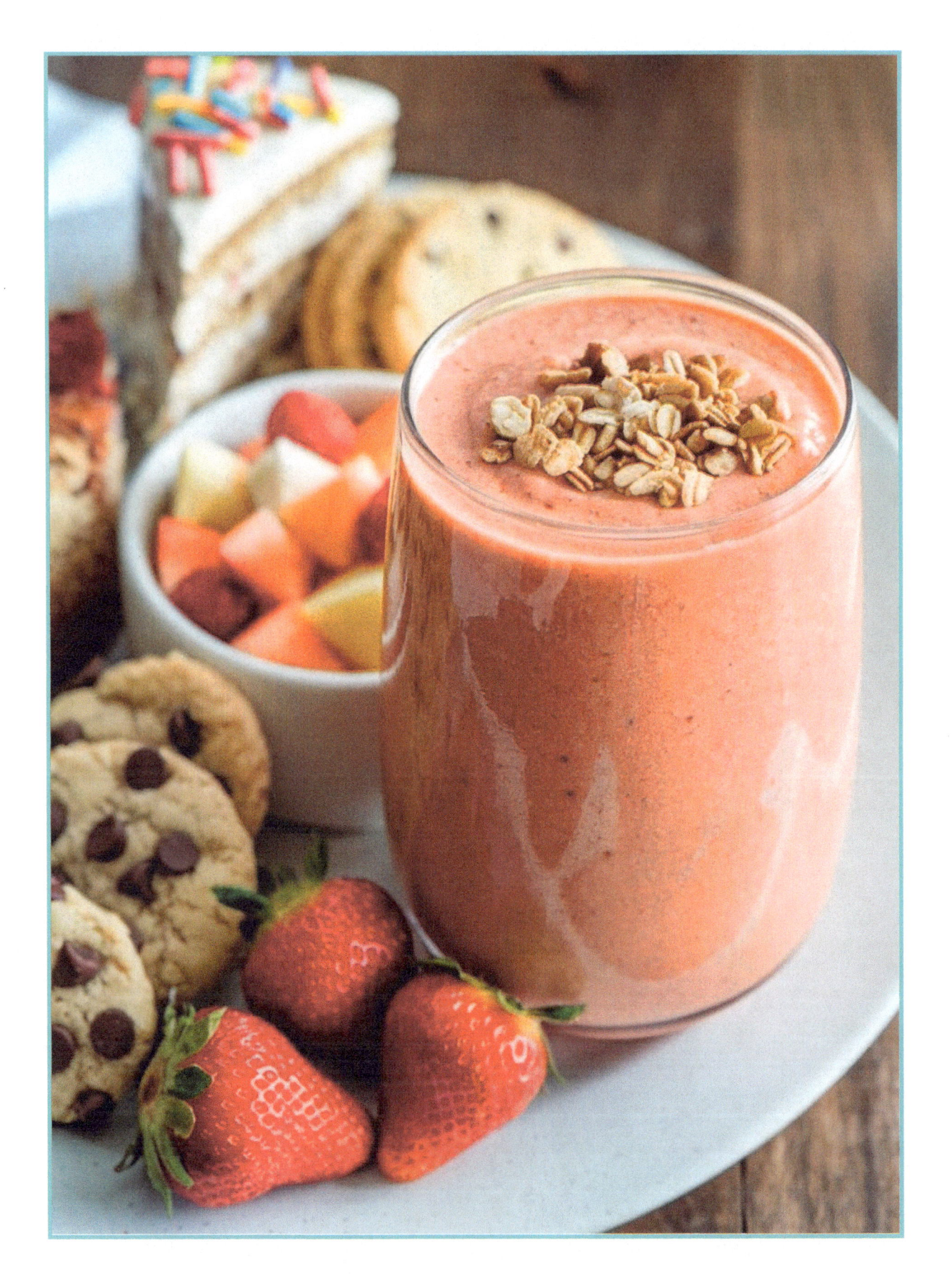

Content

Introduction 6
   1. What is Metabolic Confusion? 7
   2. Understanding Endomorph Body Type 9
   3. How This Diet Helps with Weight Loss & Energy 11
   4. Calorie Cycling Explained 15

Part I: Metabolic Confusion Basics 19
   1. Key Principles of the Diet 19
   2. Macronutrients and Your Endomorph Body 23
   3. Personalizing Your Meal Plan 28

Part II: Meal Planning 34
   1. Creating Your Meal Plan 34
   2. Calorie Cycling Tips 36
   3. Portion Control and Tracking 38
   4. Whole Foods 40

Part III: Tailored Meal Plans 42
   1. Week 1: Low-Carb Kickstart 42
   2. Week 2: Protein + Moderate Carbs 44
   3. Week 3: Carb Reintroduction 46
   4. 4, 6, and 8-Week Meal Plans 48

Part IV: Recipes 52
   1. Breakfasts: Energizing Options 52
   2. Lunches: Satisfying Meals 58

3. Dinners: Low-Calorie Recipes..65
4. Snacks: Healthy, Metabolism-Boosting...69
5. Smoothies: Quick & Nutritious..73
6. Desserts: Sweet and Supportive...77

Part V: Exercise & Lifestyle 83
1. Best Workouts for Endomorph Women...83
2. Lifestyle Tips: Sleep, Stress, Hydration...86
3. Tracking Progress & Staying Motivated...88

Part VI: Troubleshooting 90
1. Overcoming Plateaus...90
2. Adjusting for Life Changes..92
3. Common Mistakes & Solutions..93

Conclusion 96

Bonus Content 97
1. Grocery List for Beginners..97
2. Meal Prep Tips..99
3. Printable Meal Plan Templates...100

6

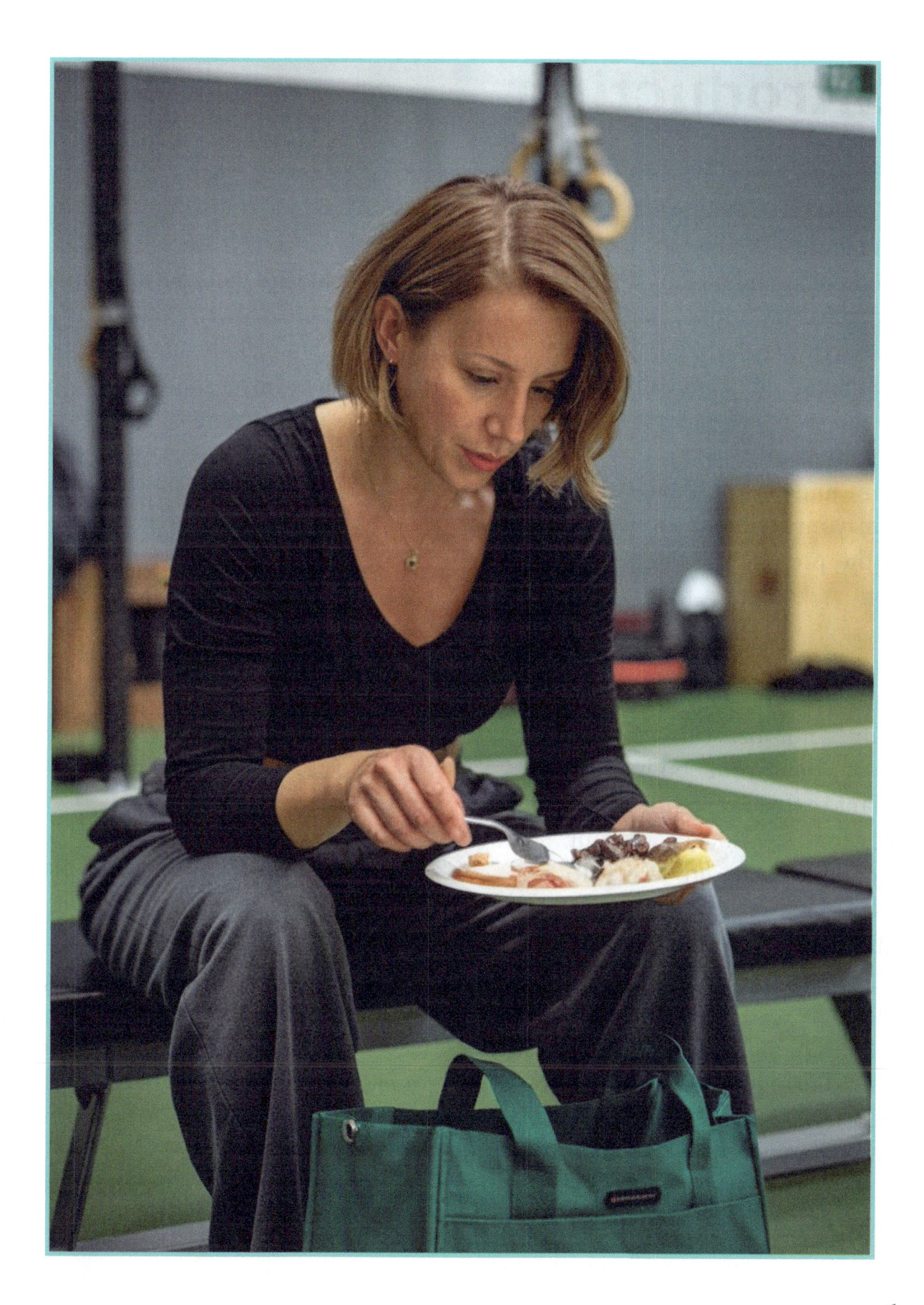

Introduction

What is Metabolic Confusion?

Metabolic Confusion is a strategic approach designed to give your metabolism a boost by alternating the number of calories you consume on a daily basis. Unlike traditional dieting, which often involves consistently restricting calories, Metabolic Confusion keeps your body guessing by switching up your caloric intake. This strategy has been shown to help enhance metabolic function, prevent plateaus, and promote sustained weight loss.

The underlying concept is that your metabolism, which is the process by which your body converts food into energy, works best when it isn't subjected to routine patterns. When you eat the same number of calories every day, your body may adapt to this constant supply, slowing down your metabolism in an effort to conserve energy. Over time, this can lead to weight loss plateaus, where you feel like you're doing everything right but aren't seeing the same results.

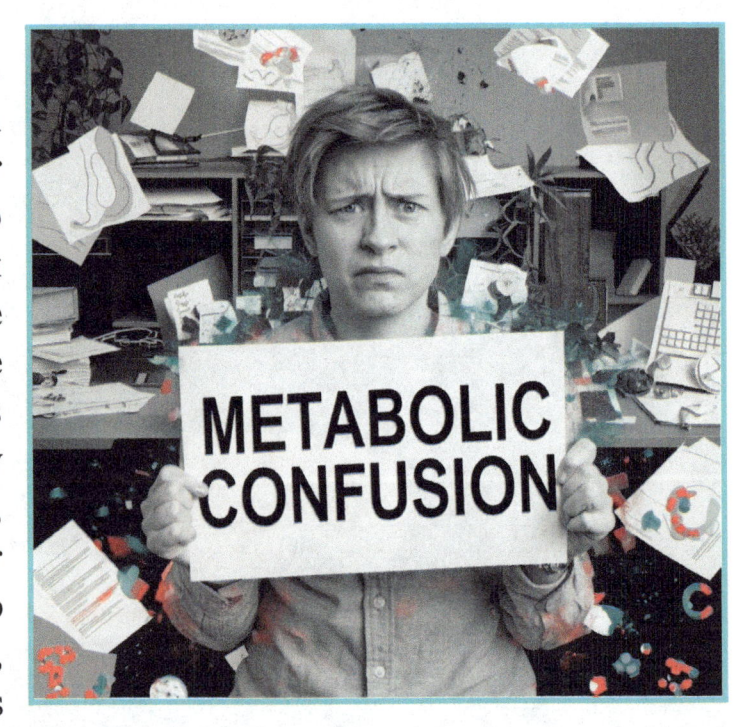

—By implementing Metabolic Confusion, we break this cycle. The goal is to give your body variety—one day you might eat a slightly higher number of calories, and the next day, you'll eat fewer. This switching up of calorie intake forces your metabolism to remain active and responsive, rather than slowing down. Your body learns to burn fat more effectively, which means you can lose weight while maintaining your energy levels.

This technique is particularly beneficial for endomorph women, who tend to have a slower metabolism and often find it more difficult to lose weight compared to other body types. Endomorphs typically carry more body fat and find that their body prefers storing energy rather than burning it. This is where Metabolic Confusion comes in handy—it prevents your metabolism from becoming sluggish and keeps your body from storing excess fat.
—The beauty of Metabolic Confusion is that it doesn't require extreme calorie restriction. Instead, it focuses on calorie cycling, which means alternating between higher and lower calorie days. This approach makes it easier to adhere to, as you aren't stuck with the same rigid eating pattern every day. Plus, you can still enjoy your favorite meals in moderation without feeling deprived or restricted.
—The key to success with Metabolic Confusion is learning how to balance your meals, ensuring that you're getting the right macronutrients (proteins, fats, and carbs) on both your high- and low-calorie days. It's not just about reducing calories; it's about timing your intake so your metabolism remains active, your energy stays high, and your body stays in fat-burning mode. This book will teach you exactly how to incorporate Metabolic Confusion into your life, with tailored meal plans, easy-to-follow recipes, and tips for success.
—In the next sections, we'll dive deeper into how Metabolic Confusion works for women with an endomorph body type and how to personalize your approach to make this diet a natural, sustainable part of your routine. You'll find everything you need right here, so let's get started and unlock your body's full potential!

Understanding Endomorph Body Type

Before diving into the specifics of how Metabolic Confusion works for your body, let's take a moment to understand the endomorph body type—the type that this cookbook is specifically designed to support.

—There are three main body types: ectomorph, mesomorph, and endomorph. Each body type has its own unique characteristics and metabolic tendencies, and knowing which one you identify with can be a game-changer when it comes to weight loss, fitness, and overall health.

—As an endomorph, you may have noticed that losing weight feels more challenging than it seems for others. You might struggle with excess fat, especially around the hips, thighs, and midsection, despite your best efforts to eat healthy and exercise. That's because endomorphs are naturally predisposed to storing fat rather than burning it, which can make weight management feel like an uphill battle.

Key Characteristics of the Endomorph Body Type:

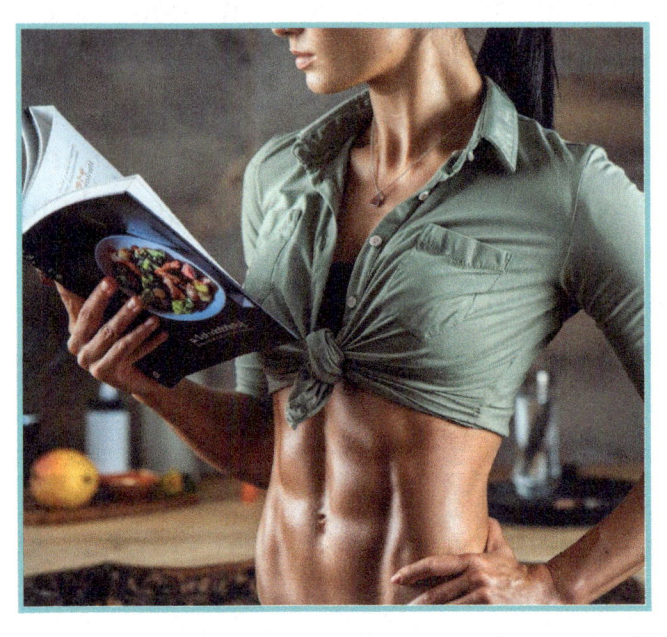

Slower Metabolism: Endomorphs tend to have a slower metabolic rate, meaning your body burns calories at a slower pace than other body types. This can make it harder to lose weight, as your body might hold onto fat more easily.

- **Increased Fat Storage**: You may notice that you gain weight more quickly than others, particularly around your midsection, hips, and thighs. Your body is more efficient at storing fat for energy, which, while beneficial in some situations, can make fat loss more difficult.
- **Naturally Larger Frame**: Endomorphs generally have a more rounded or fuller physique, with wider hips and a more solid build. While this doesn't necessarily mean you're unhealthy, it does indicate that your body tends to store fat rather than burn it.
- **Difficulty Losing Weight**: While endomorphs can gain muscle relatively easily, losing fat is often much more challenging. This is due to a combination of genetics and a slower metabolism, which means it's crucial to approach weight loss strategically.

Why Endomorphs Struggle with Weight Loss:

When you have a slower metabolism, your body uses energy more slowly, and the process of burning calories becomes less efficient. If you eat the same amount of food as someone with a faster metabolism, your body may not be able to use all those calories right away. Instead, they are stored as fat, making weight loss more difficult.

—Additionally, endomorphs often experience greater fluctuations in energy levels, which can make it harder to maintain an active lifestyle. You might find yourself feeling tired or sluggish, even if you're eating well and exercising regularly. This is another challenge that Metabolic Confusion can help address, as it not only supports fat loss but can also help regulate your energy levels throughout the day.

How Metabolic Confusion Works for Endomorphs

Metabolic Confusion works beautifully for the endomorph body type because it keeps your metabolism from slowing down. By cycling between higher and lower calorie days, Metabolic Confusion tricks your body into constantly burning fat. This strategy helps you avoid the plateau effect that often happens when following a traditional calorie-restricted diet.

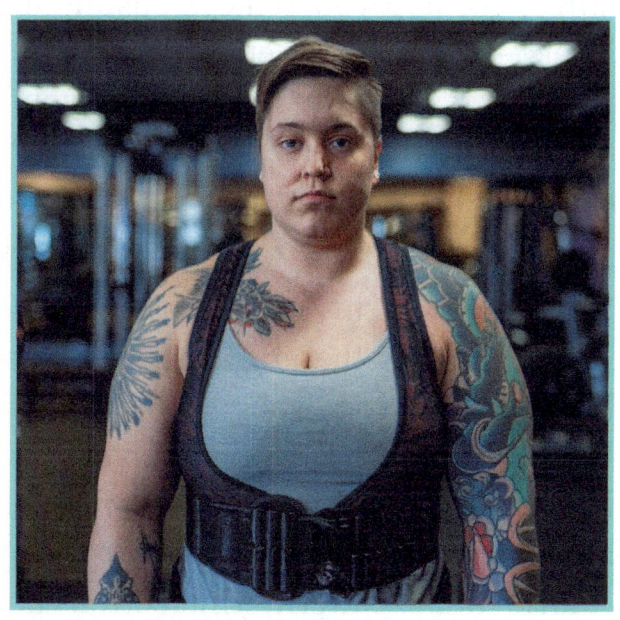

—Incorporating Metabolic Confusion into your lifestyle can help your body shift from a fat-storing mode to a fat-burning mode, which is exactly what endomorphs need. By balancing your calorie intake and ensuring that you're getting the right macronutrients at the right times, you can start to see changes in both your body composition and energy levels.

—This cookbook is all about giving you the tools to balance your meals, understand your body's needs, and boost your metabolism. Together, we'll

develop a personalized approach that works with your natural body type, helping you achieve your goals without the struggle.
—In the following sections, I'll show you exactly how to tailor your meal plans and make Metabolic Confusion work for you, so you can unlock your body's full potential and start seeing results that you can feel proud of!

How This Diet Helps with Weight Loss & Energy

One of the most powerful aspects of the Metabolic Confusion Diet is its ability to help you achieve sustainable weight loss and boost your energy levels—especially for endomorph women. This diet doesn't just aim to shed pounds; it's designed to support your body in a way that helps it function optimally, so you feel your best, both inside and out. Let me show you exactly how this approach can work wonders for you.

1. Boosts Your Metabolism:

When it comes to weight loss, your metabolism is everything. Think of your metabolism as the engine that drives the calorie-burning process in your body. For endomorphs, metabolism tends to be slower, which makes it harder to burn calories effectively. The beauty of Metabolic Confusion lies in its ability to "wake up" your metabolism. By alternating between higher- and lower-calorie days, you prevent your body from adapting to a single calorie intake pattern, which often causes your metabolism to slow down.
—When you switch up your calorie intake regularly, your body remains in a state of "confusion," forcing it to continue burning calories at a higher rate. This keeps your metabolism running at full speed, burning more fat and preventing plateaus, so you can continue losing weight even when things seem to stall on traditional diets.

2. Prevents Fat Storage:

One of the biggest challenges for endomorphs is the tendency to store fat, especially around the midsection, hips, and thighs. When your metabolism slows down, your body is more likely to store excess calories as fat instead of using them for energy. But by following a Metabolic Confusion plan, you can avoid this problem. The alternating calorie intake prevents your body from entering a state of "survival mode," where it stores fat to prepare for potential scarcity.

—On high-calorie days, your body uses those calories for energy, muscle repair, and growth. On low-calorie days, it taps into stored fat as a fuel source, promoting fat loss. The combination of high and low-calorie days ensures that your body is always using energy efficiently, avoiding fat storage, and helping you lose weight in a sustainable way.

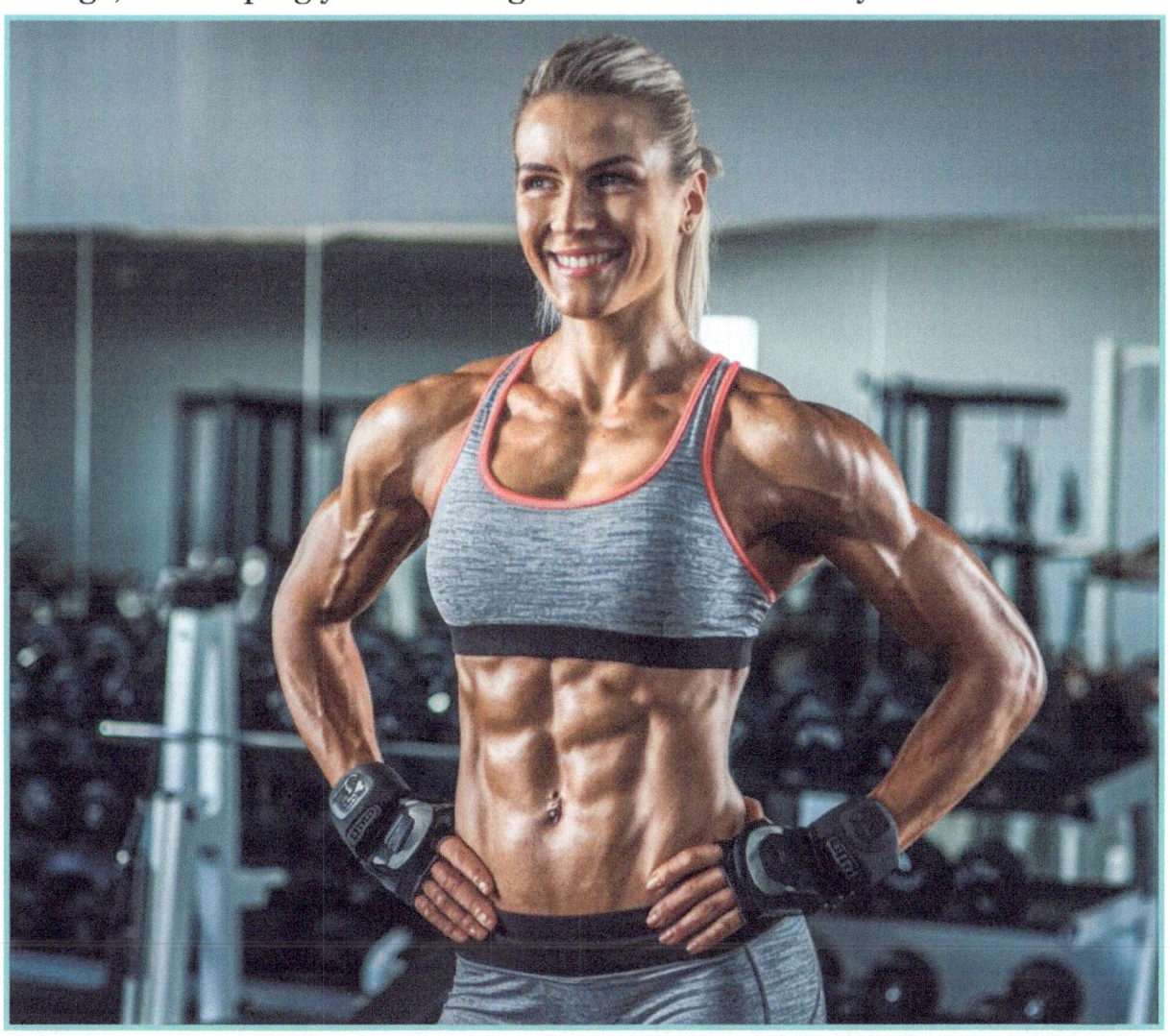

3. Balanced Energy Levels Throughout the Day:

It's so frustrating to feel sluggish and fatigued, especially when you're doing everything right with your diet and exercise. For endomorphs, this can be a frequent issue because of the slower metabolism and the difficulty your body faces when processing food. Metabolic Confusion helps you tackle this problem head-on by balancing your energy needs.

—On high-calorie days, your body receives the fuel it needs to power through your workouts and your day. These days help replenish glycogen stores in your muscles, which is your body's primary source of energy for high-intensity activities. On low-calorie days, your body learns to tap into fat stores for energy, giving you the perfect balance of fuel for daily activities without feeling sluggish or deprived.

—By cycling between these days, you avoid the blood sugar spikes and crashes that often occur on restrictive diets, ensuring that your energy remains stable throughout the day. Whether it's for work, exercise, or everyday tasks, you'll feel more energized and focused without the energy dips that leave you feeling exhausted.

4. Keeps You Feeling Full and Satisfied:

One of the reasons that traditional low-calorie diets fail for many people is because they leave you feeling hungry and deprived. When you're constantly in a calorie deficit, it can be tough to stay motivated and stick with your plan long-term. But Metabolic Confusion is different. The alternating calorie intake ensures that you don't experience extreme hunger on your low-calorie days.

—On higher-calorie days, you get the satisfaction of eating more food, while still supporting fat loss. You're still consuming nutrient-dense foods, but you're doing so in a way that keeps you feeling full, satisfied, and energized. This helps you avoid overeating, binge eating, or falling off track because of hunger or cravings.

5. Improves Fat-Burning Efficiency:

One of the standout benefits of Metabolic Confusion is that it doesn't just focus on weight loss as a one-time thing; it encourages your body to learn how to burn fat more efficiently. When you follow this approach over time, your body becomes better at utilizing fat as an energy source, even on days when you're consuming fewer calories. This means you can continue to lose fat, even when you're not always in a major calorie deficit.

By incorporating the right foods, balanced macronutrients, and the strategic calorie cycling of Metabolic Confusion, your body learns to be more efficient at burning fat—whether you're at rest, working, or exercising. This fat-burning efficiency is what helps you maintain your results long-term, so you don't just lose weight; you transform your metabolism into a fat-burning machine.

Calorie Cycling Explained

One of the key pillars of the Metabolic Confusion Diet is calorie cycling, and it's one of the most powerful strategies for achieving sustainable weight loss while maintaining high energy levels. If you've ever tried dieting before, you might be familiar with the concept of calorie restriction—but calorie cycling takes that idea to the next level by allowing you to switch up your calorie intake on different days. This keeps your metabolism running efficiently, prevents plateaus, and helps you burn fat while still fueling your body with the nutrients it needs.

Let me break down how calorie cycling works and how it can help you on your weight loss journey.

What is Calorie Cycling?

Calorie cycling is exactly what it sounds like: alternating between higher-calorie days and lower-calorie days. Unlike traditional diets that require a consistent calorie deficit (where you eat fewer calories than you burn every single day), calorie cycling allows for flexibility. Some days, you'll eat more; other days, you'll eat less. The idea is to "trick" your metabolism into staying active and efficient, which helps you burn fat more effectively.

—By shifting between different calorie intake levels, you can maintain a steady metabolic rate, prevent your body from adapting to one routine, and encourage it to burn fat without the negative effects of extreme calorie restriction. It's about giving your body what it needs to stay energized and healthy, while still promoting weight loss.

How Does Calorie Cycling Work?

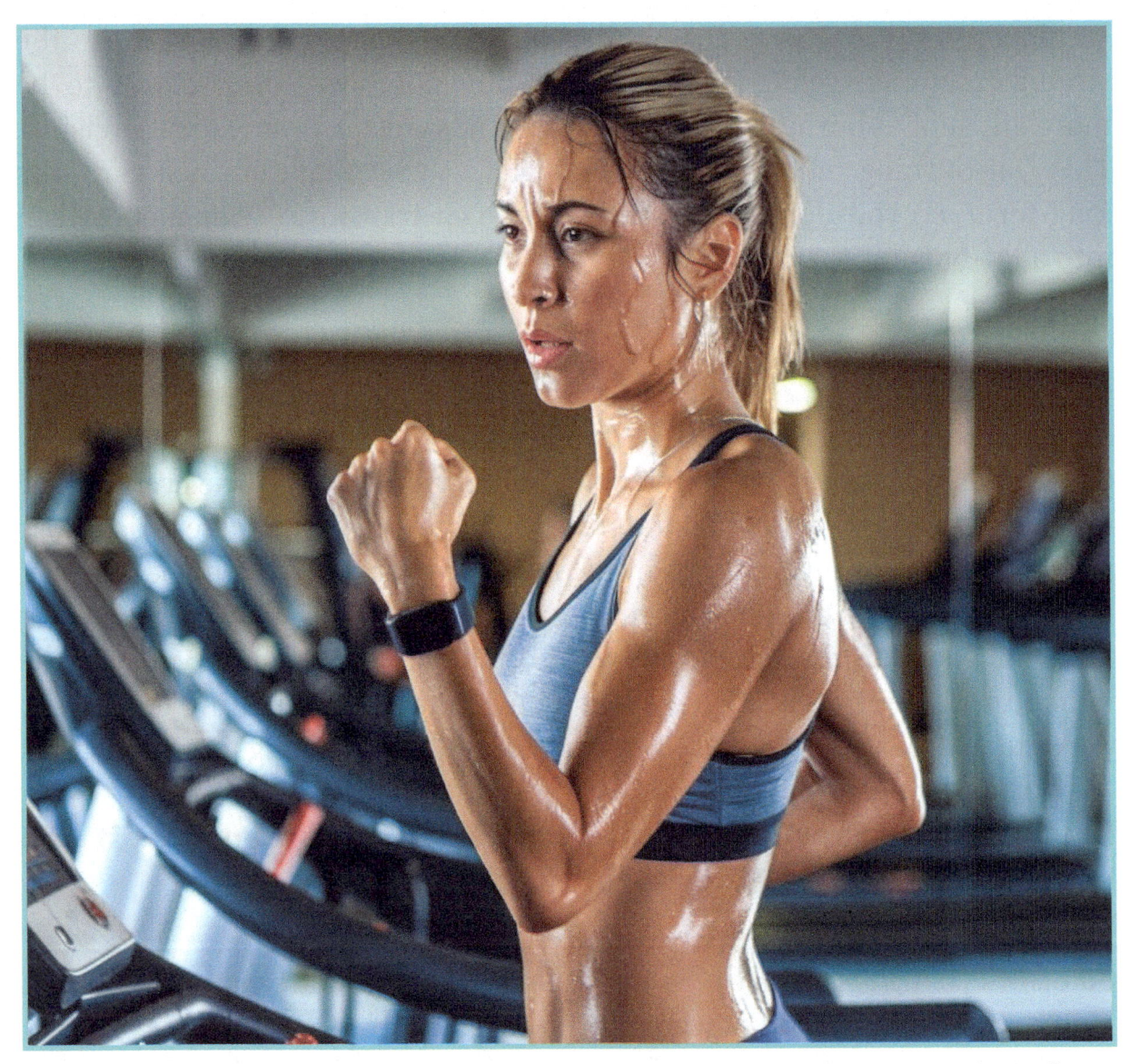

When you follow a calorie cycling approach, you don't have to worry about sticking to a strict low-calorie routine day after day. Instead, you alternate your intake. Here's how it works:

- **Higher-Calorie Days**: These days are designed to give your metabolism a boost. You'll eat more calories than usual, typically from nutrient-dense foods like lean proteins, healthy fats, and complex carbohydrates. On these days, your body is replenishing its energy stores and ensuring you have enough fuel for your workouts, muscle recovery, and daily activities. These higher-calorie days are key for preventing metabolic slowdown and keeping you from feeling deprived.

- **Lower-Calorie Days**: These days, you reduce your calorie intake, typically by cutting back on carbohydrates or fats. This allows your body to tap into stored fat for energy, promoting fat loss. Because your body has already been fueled on higher-calorie days, it's not in starvation mode. Instead, it switches to burning fat more efficiently for fuel. Lower-calorie days help you create a calorie deficit in a way that's manageable and sustainable, without triggering the hunger and fatigue that often accompany traditional dieting.

Why Does Calorie Cycling Work?

Prevents Metabolic Slowdown: One of the biggest challenges with consistent calorie restriction is that your metabolism can slow down over time. When your body gets used to eating fewer calories, it tries to conserve energy by reducing its metabolic rate. This can lead to a plateau, where weight loss stalls despite sticking to a low-calorie diet. Calorie cycling prevents this by constantly "shocking" your system. On higher-calorie days, your metabolism gets a boost, while on lower-calorie days, it stays active, ensuring your fat-burning abilities remain intact.

Keeps Your Body Guessing: When your body knows it's getting the same number of calories every day, it starts to adapt to that routine. This can make fat loss harder over time, as your body becomes more efficient at storing fat instead of burning it. By cycling your calories, you prevent this adaptation. Each day is different, and your metabolism doesn't know what to expect, which means it continues to burn fat more effectively.

- **Improves Fat Burning**: On lower-calorie days, your body has to turn to its fat stores for energy. This encourages fat loss without requiring you to starve yourself or dramatically restrict your food intake. By alternating with higher-calorie days, you can ensure that your body has enough energy to keep up with your workouts, daily activities, and overall metabolic needs.
- **Supports Energy Levels**: One of the biggest concerns with dieting is the risk of feeling drained and sluggish, especially if you're constantly in a calorie deficit. With calorie cycling, you can avoid those energy dips. On your higher-calorie days, you'll have the energy you need to fuel workouts, perform daily tasks, and feel your best. On

lower-calorie days, you'll still be able to function without feeling overly fatigued, thanks to the careful balance of energy intake over time.

How to Implement Calorie Cycling in Your Diet:

Calorie cycling isn't complicated, but it does require some planning. Here's a simple way to get started:

- **Set Your Daily Calorie Needs**: The first step is to determine how many calories you need to maintain your current weight. There are many tools available online to help you calculate your Total Daily Energy Expenditure (TDEE), which tells you how many calories you burn on a daily basis based on your activity level.
- **Establish Your Calorie Cycling Pattern**: A common approach is to have a 2:1 or 3:1 ratio, where you alternate between two or three low-calorie days and one higher-calorie day. For example, you might eat at a calorie deficit on Monday, Wednesday, and Friday, and then eat at maintenance or slightly above maintenance on Tuesday and Thursday. Your weekend might include a higher-calorie day as well.
- **Choose Your Foods Wisely**: While calorie cycling allows for flexibility, the quality of your food choices is still important. Focus on nutrient-dense foods, like lean proteins, healthy fats, and whole grains, that will provide lasting energy and support your metabolism. On higher-calorie days, you can add more healthy carbs or fats, and on lower-calorie days, you'll want to focus on protein and vegetables to keep your metabolism active while controlling your calorie intake.
- **Listen to Your Body**: Pay attention to how your body responds to calorie cycling. You may need to adjust your calorie intake or cycling schedule based on how you feel, your progress, and your energy levels. The goal is to find a balance that works for you, allowing you to lose weight while still feeling energized and nourished.

Calorie cycling is a simple yet powerful tool that can help endomorphs—like yourself—accelerate fat loss while maintaining energy levels. By cycling your calorie intake between higher and lower days, you can keep your metabolism working efficiently, avoid plateaus, and make your weight loss journey more sustainable. Plus, it offers the flexibility to enjoy a variety of foods without feeling deprived.

Part I: Metabolic Confusion Basics

Key Principles of the Diet

Welcome to the first step in your Metabolic Confusion journey! In this section, we're going to explore the key principles behind this diet and how they work together to help you achieve weight loss, boost energy, and improve overall well-being. Understanding these foundational principles will not only give you the knowledge you need to succeed but also empower you to make the best choices for your body.

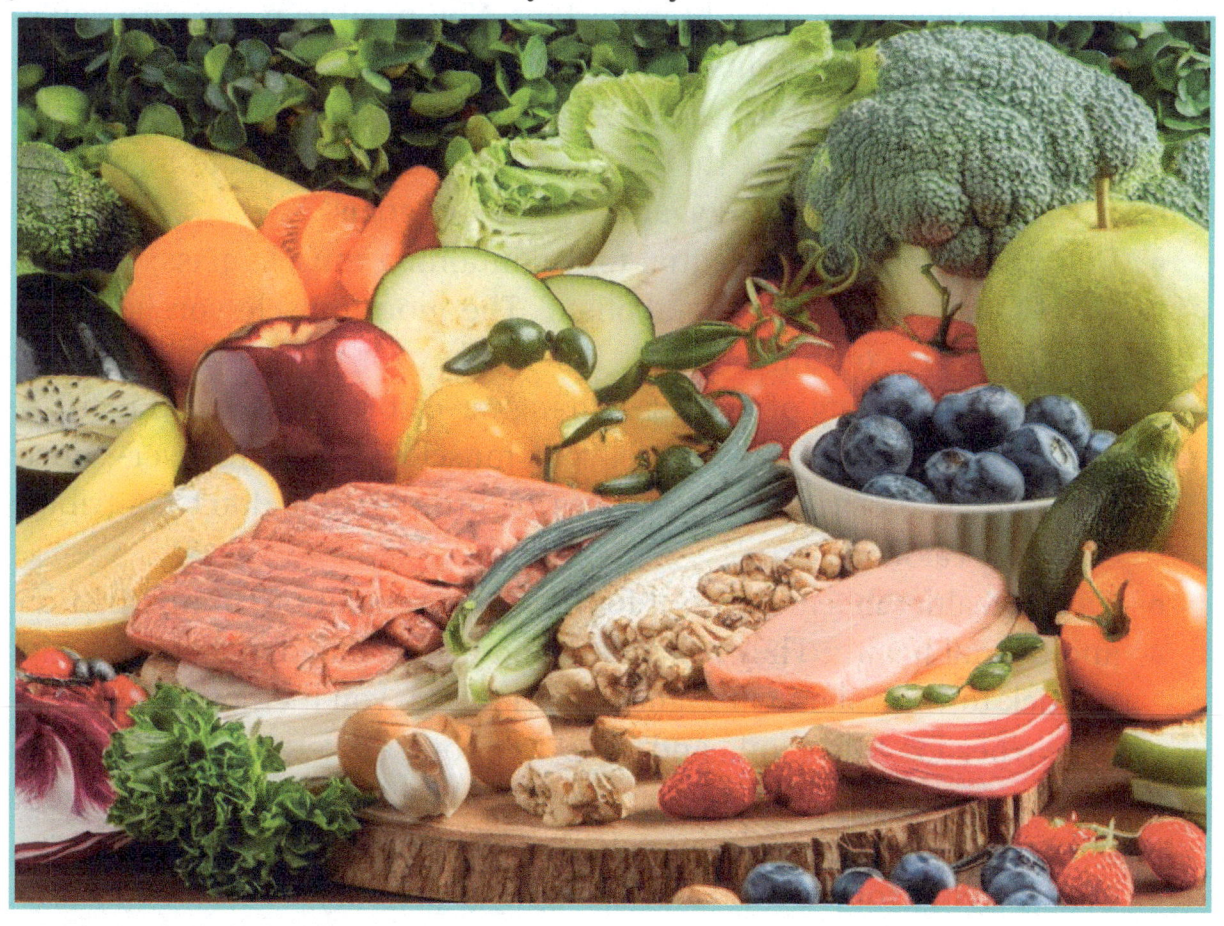

1. Calorie Cycling:

At the core of the Metabolic Confusion Diet is calorie cycling, which we discussed earlier. This principle is all about alternating between higher-calorie and lower-calorie days. By doing so, your body never gets used to a single routine, and your metabolism stays active, burning calories efficiently. This keeps you from hitting weight loss plateaus, as your body is constantly adjusting and adapting. It also allows you to enjoy more food on certain days without compromising your progress.

—This approach is particularly helpful for endomorphs, as it keeps the metabolism firing on all cylinders, even when you're eating fewer calories on certain days. Calorie cycling prevents the dreaded "starvation mode" that can occur with traditional diets, ensuring your body doesn't slow down its fat-burning process.

2. Macronutrient Balance

While calorie cycling is the main focus of the Metabolic Confusion Diet, macronutrient balance is equally important. You need to make sure you're getting the right mix of proteins, fats, and carbohydrates to support both fat loss and muscle maintenance. Each macronutrient plays a unique role in the body, and understanding their impact will help you create meals that support your metabolism, energy, and weight loss goals.

- **Proteins**: Protein is essential for maintaining muscle mass, which is important for boosting metabolism. The more muscle you have, the more calories you burn at rest. It's also key for repairing tissues and promoting a feeling of fullness. On higher-calorie days, you'll increase your protein intake to help fuel your muscles, while on lower-calorie days, you'll focus on lean sources of protein that don't contribute excessive calories.
- **Fats**: Healthy fats are crucial for hormone regulation, brain function, and overall health. They also help keep you satisfied, making it easier to stick to your plan. On higher-calorie days, you'll enjoy healthy fats like avocados, olive oil, and nuts to provide sustained energy. On lower-calorie days, the key is moderation—aiming for small portions of healthy fats that won't put you over your calorie limit.
- **Carbohydrates**: Carbs are the body's primary source of energy. They provide fuel for workouts, muscle recovery, and daily activities.

When calorie cycling, you'll adjust your carbohydrate intake based on the day's calorie requirements. On high-calorie days, you'll increase complex carbs like whole grains, sweet potatoes, and legumes to replenish glycogen stores and fuel your body. On low-calorie days, you'll opt for low-glycemic carbs such as leafy greens, cauliflower, and zucchini, which provide essential nutrients without the calorie load.

3. Flexibility and Sustainability

One of the most appealing aspects of the Metabolic Confusion Diet is its flexibility. Unlike restrictive diets that require you to follow rigid rules, Metabolic Confusion allows for a more varied approach, giving you the freedom to enjoy different types of foods while still staying on track with your weight loss goals. This flexibility makes it easier to stick with the diet long-term, as you're not depriving yourself of food you enjoy.
—Metabolic Confusion isn't about eating less—it's about eating smart. The focus is on quality nutrition and strategic planning. The cycling between high- and low-calorie days provides structure, but you can still make choices that work for your lifestyle, tastes, and preferences.
—Sustainability is key. This diet doesn't demand drastic cuts or extreme measures. It's designed to fit into your life, helping you make healthier food choices without the constant pressure of counting every calorie. Instead, it's about finding a balance that feels natural, maintains energy, and supports weight loss over time.

4. Personalized Approach

This diet is all about personalization. Everyone's body responds differently to food, which is why Metabolic Confusion gives you the tools to adjust the diet to suit your unique needs. As an endomorph, you'll learn how to tailor the number of calories, macronutrients, and meal timing to your individual metabolism and goals. There is no one-size-fits-all solution here—this diet encourages you to find what works best for you.
—You'll also be able to modify your approach based on changes in your lifestyle, activity level, and progress. Whether you're more active some days or you want to enjoy a meal out with friends, Metabolic Confusion allows you to make adjustments as needed. The key is to always keep your

metabolism guessing and your body fueled with the right balance of nutrients.

5. No Deprivation—Just Smart Eating
One of the biggest frustrations with traditional diets is the feeling of deprivation. You often have to sacrifice the foods you love in exchange for restrictive eating habits. But Metabolic Confusion is different. This diet encourages you to enjoy the foods you love, while still making smart, informed choices.

—Higher-calorie days offer a chance to indulge in more satisfying meals without guilt. Think of these days as an opportunity to enjoy your favorite foods in moderation. The flexibility of the diet ensures that you're never stuck eating bland, boring meals. On the flip side, lower-calorie days help you stay on track with fat loss, ensuring that you still get to see the results you're working hard for.

—'With Metabolic Confusion, you'll learn how to maintain a healthy balance between enjoying your food and staying on course with your goals.

Macronutrients and Your Endomorph Body

Now that you've learned the basics of the Metabolic Confusion Diet, it's time to dive deeper into how macronutrients—the three key components of every meal (proteins, fats, and carbohydrates)—play a critical role in your journey to weight loss and increased energy. Understanding how to balance these macronutrients is especially important for endomorph women, as your body has unique needs when it comes to how it processes and utilizes food.

—So let's break down each macronutrient, how it impacts your metabolism, and how to tailor your intake to support your weight loss and energy goals.

1. Protein: The Muscle-Builder and Fat-Burner
Protein is one of the most important macronutrients for your endomorph body. If you've ever wondered why protein is so emphasized in most fitness and weight loss plans, it's because of the many vital functions it serves in the body. For endomorphs, who often struggle with maintaining a lean

physique, protein becomes even more essential for building muscle, keeping metabolism active, and supporting fat loss.

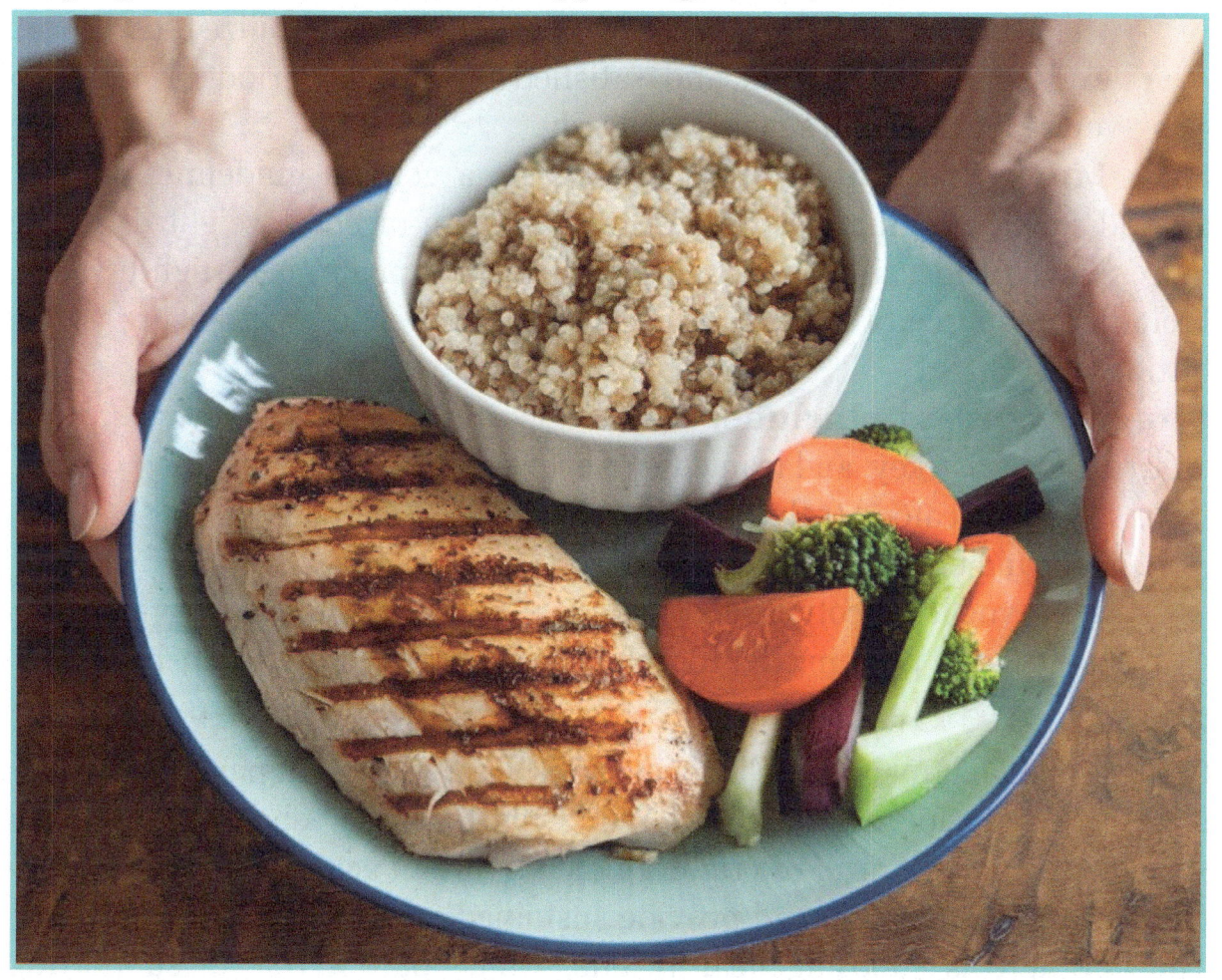

Why Protein Is Important for Endomorphs:
- **Builds and Repairs Muscle**: Protein is key for muscle repair and growth. Since endomorphs typically have a naturally higher body fat percentage and might find it harder to burn fat, having more lean muscle mass helps increase your resting metabolic rate. The more muscle you have, the more calories you burn—even when you're not exercising.
- **Boosts Metabolism**: Your metabolism works harder to break down protein than it does with carbs or fats. This means that eating more protein can help keep your metabolism fired up, which is crucial for fat loss. Protein helps promote the thermic effect of food (TEF), which is the energy your body uses to digest, absorb, and metabolize food.

- **Keeps You Full Longer**: Protein is also very satiating. As someone with an endomorph body type, it's essential to avoid hunger cravings, which can often lead to overeating. Protein helps stabilize blood sugar levels, keeping you full and satisfied for longer periods of time, so you're less likely to snack mindlessly.

How Much Protein Do You Need? As a general guideline, aim for around 1.2 to 1.6 grams of protein per kilogram of body weight. If you're more active or focusing on muscle-building, you might need slightly more. Including a source of protein in every meal and snack will ensure you're hitting your goals.

Protein Sources to Include:
1. Chicken, turkey, and lean cuts of beef or pork
2. Fish and seafood (salmon, tuna, shrimp)
3. Eggs and egg whites
4. Greek yogurt or cottage cheese
5. Plant-based proteins (lentils, chickpeas, quinoa, tofu, tempeh)

2. Fat: The Hormone Regulator and Energy Source

Contrary to what many people believe, fats are an essential part of a healthy diet—especially for endomorphs. While it's true that endomorphs often struggle with fat storage, the right kinds of fats can actually help your body burn fat more efficiently and provide sustained energy throughout the day. The key here is choosing healthy fats, which play a role in supporting hormone function, brain health, and fat metabolism.

Why Fats Are Important for Endomorphs:

- **Regulates Hormones**: Fats are essential for hormone production, including those that control appetite, metabolism, and fat storage. Proper fat intake ensures your hormones are balanced, which helps your body maintain an efficient metabolism and manage hunger.
- **Provides Long-Lasting Energy**: Unlike carbohydrates, which provide quick bursts of energy and can leave you feeling tired once they've been burned, fats offer a steady release of energy. Healthy fats help fuel your workouts, daily activities, and even your brain functions, without the spikes and crashes associated with high-carb diets.

- **Supports Fat Burning**: Healthy fats, particularly those found in omega-3 fatty acids, can aid in fat burning by promoting fat oxidation (the process your body uses to burn fat for fuel). This is particularly important for endomorphs who want to keep fat storage at bay while still maintaining energy for their workouts and daily routines.

How Much Fat Do You Need? Fat intake should make up about 25-35% of your total daily calories. Aim to focus on healthy fats and incorporate them strategically on high-calorie days to maintain energy levels and prevent fat storage.

Healthy Fat Sources to Include:
1. Avocados and avocado oil
2. Nuts (almonds, walnuts, cashews) and seeds (chia, flax, pumpkin)
3. Fatty fish (salmon, mackerel, sardines)
4. Olive oil and coconut oil
5. Nut butters (peanut butter, almond butter)

3. Carbohydrates: The Fuel for Your Workouts and Daily Life

Carbohydrates are the body's primary source of energy, and while some people fear carbs, they're actually a vital part of a balanced diet—especially for endomorphs who may need a little extra energy for their workouts. Carbs fuel your muscles, replenish glycogen stores, and give you the stamina you need to power through the day. The trick for endomorphs is choosing the right types of carbohydrates and consuming them in the right amounts.

Why Carbs Are Important for Endomorphs:

- **Energy for Workouts**: Carbs are your body's go-to source of energy for high-intensity exercise. For endomorphs, who may find that their body doesn't burn fat as efficiently, consuming the right types of carbs ensures you have the energy to engage in fat-burning workouts that support weight loss.
- **Helps with Muscle Recovery**: After intense physical activity, carbs help replenish glycogen stores in your muscles, allowing for

quicker recovery and preventing fatigue. This helps you stay energized and motivated for your next workout.
- **Regulates Blood Sugar**: Whole carbs, especially those with a low glycemic index (like sweet potatoes and whole grains), help stabilize blood sugar levels, preventing the spikes and crashes that can lead to cravings and overeating.

How Much Carbohydrate Do You Need? Carbs should make up about 40-50% of your total daily calories. On higher-calorie days, you can increase your carb intake slightly to replenish glycogen and fuel your workouts. On lower-calorie days, you can reduce carb intake while still including plenty of fiber-rich, nutrient-dense options.

Healthy Carbohydrate Sources to Include:
1. Sweet potatoes, butternut squash, and other root vegetables
2. Whole grains (quinoa, brown rice, oats, barley)
3. Legumes (beans, lentils, chickpeas)
4. Leafy greens and non-starchy vegetables (spinach, kale, broccoli)
5. Fruits (berries, apples, pears)

Balancing your macronutrients—protein, fat, and carbohydrates—is key for your endomorph body to thrive on the Metabolic Confusion Diet. Protein supports muscle building and metabolism, healthy fats regulate hormones and energy, and carbs fuel your workouts and recovery. By customizing your intake based on the needs of your body, you can help boost your metabolism, increase energy levels, and achieve your weight loss goals.

Personalizing Your Meal Plan

One of the greatest advantages of the Metabolic Confusion Diet is that it allows for a highly personalized approach. There's no one-size-fits-all plan here—your body is unique, and your meal plan should reflect your individual needs, preferences, and goals. The key to success is understanding your metabolism, adjusting your calories and macronutrients accordingly, and finding a rhythm that works for you.

—Let's dive into how to personalize your Metabolic Confusion meal plan so it aligns with your body type, activity level, and weight loss goals, ensuring you can stay energized, satisfied, and on track.

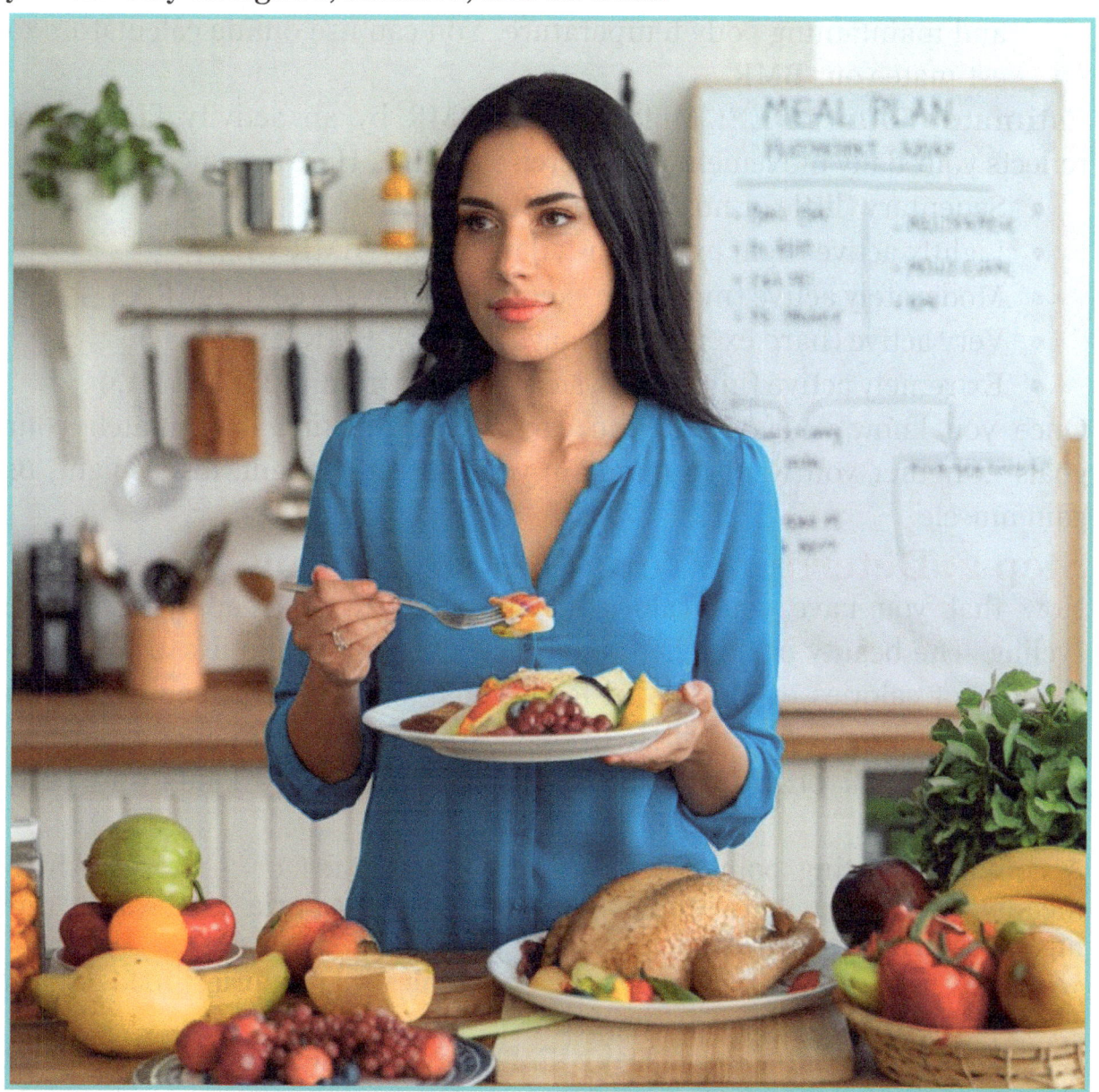

Step 1: Understand Your Calorie Needs

The first step in creating a personalized meal plan is determining how many calories your body needs. This is based on your Total Daily Energy Expenditure (TDEE), which accounts for your basal metabolic rate (BMR)—the calories your body needs at rest—and the calories burned through physical activity.

To get started:
- **Calculate Your BMR**: This is the amount of energy (calories) your body needs to perform basic functions like breathing, digesting food, and maintaining body temperature. You can use online calculators to estimate your BMR.

Estimate Your TDEE: Multiply your BMR by an activity factor that reflects your daily movement and exercise routine. Here's a quick guide:
- Sedentary (little or no exercise): BMR x 1.2
- Lightly active (light exercise 1-3 days/week): BMR x 1.375
- Moderately active (moderate exercise 3-5 days/week): BMR x 1.55
- Very active (hard exercise 6-7 days a week): BMR x 1.725
- Extremely active (intense physical labor or training): BMR x 1.9

Once you know your TDEE, you can begin adjusting it to match your goals—whether you want to maintain your current weight, lose weight, or gain muscle.

Step 2: Determine Your Calorie Cycling Pattern

Now that you have your calorie needs, you can start applying calorie cycling. The beauty of this diet is that you don't have to stick to the same number of calories every day. Instead, you'll alternate between high- and low-calorie days, which will help keep your metabolism in fat-burning mode while still providing enough energy for your workouts and daily activities.

A common starting point for calorie cycling is a 2:1 or 3:1 ratio, which means alternating between two or three low-calorie days and one higher-calorie day. **For example:**
- Day 1 & 2 (Low-Calorie Days): Consume fewer calories, focusing on lean protein and vegetables.
- Day 3 (Higher-Calorie Day): Eat more calories, with a balance of healthy carbs, protein, and fats to replenish your energy and muscle glycogen.

You can adjust the number of high-calorie days based on your activity level and how your body responds. On days when you have intense workouts or need extra energy, increase your calories slightly. On rest days, reduce your intake to create a calorie deficit for fat loss.

Step 3: Balance Your Macronutrients

Now that you know how many calories you should be eating on high- and low-calorie days, it's time to look at your macronutrient breakdown—the balance of protein, fats, and carbohydrates—for each meal. This will ensure that your body is getting the nutrients it needs to function optimally and support your weight loss goals.

- **On High-Calorie Days**: Focus on providing your body with a well-rounded mix of protein, healthy fats, and carbs to replenish energy stores and fuel your muscles. You'll want to prioritize nutrient-dense, whole foods that provide vitamins, minerals, and fiber.

Example macronutrient breakdown for high-calorie days:
- Protein: 30-35%
- Carbohydrates: 40-45%
- Fats: 25-30%

On Low-Calorie Days: Reduce your carb intake slightly while maintaining a focus on protein and healthy fats. This helps promote fat burning without causing extreme hunger or fatigue. You'll still need enough protein to support muscle maintenance and healthy fat intake to regulate hormones and keep your energy levels stable.

Example macronutrient breakdown for low-calorie days:
- Protein: 35-40%
- Carbohydrates: 20-25%
- Fats: 35-40%

Remember that these are general guidelines. Depending on your individual needs, you can adjust your macronutrient ratios to better suit your preferences or lifestyle.

Step 4: Plan Your Meals Around Whole Foods

When personalizing your meal plan, it's important to prioritize whole, nutrient-dense foods over processed or refined options. Whole foods are packed with vitamins, minerals, and fiber, which support your metabolism, energy, and overall health. Eating a variety of colorful fruits and vegetables, lean proteins, and healthy fats ensures you get the right balance of nutrients to help your body function optimally.

Focus on including these food groups:
- Lean Proteins: Chicken, turkey, fish, eggs, tofu, and legumes.
- Healthy Fats: Avocados, olive oil, coconut oil, nuts, and seeds.
- Complex Carbohydrates: Sweet potatoes, quinoa, brown rice, oats, and whole grains.
- Vegetables and Greens: Kale, spinach, broccoli, cauliflower, zucchini, and peppers.
- Fruits: Berries, apples, pears, and citrus fruits for fiber and antioxidants.

Planning your meals around whole foods ensures that you're not only getting the right macronutrient balance but also nourishing your body with the essential vitamins and minerals it needs to stay healthy and strong.

Step 5: Monitor Your Progress and Adjust

Personalizing your meal plan is an ongoing process. Once you start following your calorie cycling plan, monitor your progress regularly. Are you losing weight at a healthy and sustainable rate? Are you feeling energized, or do you need to adjust your calorie intake or macronutrient balance?

Here are a few tips for fine-tuning your meal plan:
- Track your meals for a few days to see if you're sticking to your calorie and macronutrient goals.
- Listen to your body—are you feeling hungry or satisfied after meals? Adjust portion sizes or add more protein or healthy fats if necessary.

Adjust as needed: If you hit a plateau or your energy levels dip, you may need to tweak your calorie intake or adjust the types of foods you're eating. Increasing your protein intake or adding more vegetables can sometimes help break through a plateau.

Step 6: Meal Prep for Success

To stay on track and avoid temptations, consider prepping your meals in advance. Meal prepping allows you to control your calorie intake, portion sizes, and macronutrient balance. Spend a day each week prepping your meals, chopping veggies, cooking proteins, and measuring out portions so you can grab and go when life gets busy.

Part II: Meal Planning

Now that you have a clear understanding of Metabolic Confusion and how it works with your endomorph body type, it's time to put the theory into practice by creating your personalized meal plan. In this section, we'll focus on how to build your meal plan around calorie cycling, giving you the flexibility to enjoy the foods you love while staying on track with your weight loss and energy goals.

—Let's dive into the steps for creating a meal plan that works for you, along with some helpful calorie cycling tips to ensure you stay energized, satisfied, and motivated.

Creating Your Meal Plan

Creating a meal plan may sound overwhelming at first, but once you break it down, it's a simple and effective way to ensure you're nourishing your body the right way. The goal is to have meals that align with your calorie needs, provide balanced macronutrients, and keep your metabolism fired up. Here's how to create your plan:

Step 1: Determine Your High- and Low-Calorie Days

First, you'll need to decide how often you want to alternate between high-calorie days and low-calorie days. Typically, a 2:1 or 3:1 ratio works well for most people, meaning you'll have two or three low-calorie days followed by one high-calorie day.

- **High-Calorie Days**: These are your "refuel" days, where you eat more calories to replenish energy stores, build muscle, and avoid metabolic slowdown. These are typically scheduled on days when you have intense workouts or need extra energy.
- **Low-Calorie Days**: On these days, you reduce your calorie intake to promote fat burning. However, the goal is not to drastically cut calories but to create a manageable deficit while still feeling full and satisfied.

Step 2: Focus on Whole Foods

When creating your meal plan, make sure to prioritize whole, nutrient-dense foods. These foods provide your body with the vitamins, minerals, and antioxidants it needs to stay healthy while keeping you feeling full and energized. Your meals should include:

- **Lean proteins: Chicken, turkey, fish, eggs, tofu, and legumes.**
- **Healthy fats**: Avocados, olive oil, nuts, and seeds.
- **Complex carbs**: Whole grains, sweet potatoes, quinoa, and oats.
- **Vegetables and greens**: Leafy greens, cruciferous vegetables, and non-starchy veggies.
- **Fruits**: Berries, apples, citrus fruits, and pears for natural sweetness and fiber.

Step 3: Portion Control and Macronutrient Balance

On high-calorie days, increase your intake of complex carbohydrates (like sweet potatoes, brown rice, and whole grains) to fuel workouts and muscle recovery, while ensuring a balance of protein and fats. On low-calorie days, focus on higher protein intake to maintain muscle and reduce carbs while still including healthy fats to keep you satisfied.

Here's an example of how to balance your macronutrients:
- High-Calorie Day: 30-35% Protein, 40-45% Carbs, 25-30% Fats
- Low-Calorie Day: 35-40% Protein, 20-25% Carbs, 35-40% Fats

Step 4: Plan Your Meals and Snacks

Now, it's time to break your meals down into individual meals and snacks.

A balanced day of eating typically consists of:
- **Breakfast**: A hearty and filling meal to kickstart your metabolism.
- **Lunch**: A balanced meal that keeps you full through the afternoon.
- **Dinner**: A lighter but still satisfying meal.
- **Snacks**: Healthy, protein-packed snacks to keep hunger at bay.

Here's a quick breakdown for each meal:
- **Breakfast**: Focus on protein (eggs, Greek yogurt) with a small portion of carbs (oats, berries) and healthy fats (avocado, nuts).

- **Lunch**: A lean protein (chicken, turkey) with a salad or veggies and a complex carb (sweet potato, quinoa).
- **Dinner**: Lean protein (fish, tofu) with a variety of non-starchy vegetables and healthy fats (olive oil, avocado).
- **Snacks**: Nuts, hard-boiled eggs, Greek yogurt, or veggies with hummus.

Step 5: Meal Prep for the Week

To make life easier, plan your meals for the week ahead and meal prep. This way, you'll have healthy, portioned meals ready to go. Meal prepping ensures that you stick to your calorie and macronutrient goals and prevents you from reaching for less nutritious options when you're in a rush.

Calorie Cycling Tips

To ensure your Metabolic Confusion journey is a success, here are some calorie cycling tips that will help you navigate your high- and low-calorie days while keeping things sustainable and enjoyable:

Tip 1: Listen to Your Body's Hunger Signals

One of the best aspects of Metabolic Confusion is its flexibility. On low-calorie days, it's important not to feel deprived. If you find yourself hungry, adjust your portions slightly or add more vegetables and protein. On high-calorie days, don't overeat just because you're "allowed" to. Focus on eating mindfully, savoring the food, and stopping when you're satisfied, not stuffed.

Tip 2: Don't Skip Your High-Calorie Days

Some people may think that skipping a high-calorie day will speed up weight loss, but this can backfire. Your metabolism needs the higher-calorie days to stay active and avoid slowing down. Skipping them can lead to muscle loss, slower metabolism, and even weight loss plateaus. Stick to your planned high-calorie days to keep your body burning fat effectively.

Tip 3: Stay Hydrated

Whether you're cycling calories or sticking to a regular routine, staying hydrated is crucial. Water helps regulate metabolism, supports digestion, and keeps your energy levels high. Drink water throughout the day and consider adding herbal teas or electrolyte-rich drinks for extra hydration.

Tip 4: Incorporate a Variety of Vegetables

On low-calorie days, make sure to load up on non-starchy vegetables. These are low in calories but high in nutrients, fiber, and volume, helping you feel full without overloading on calories. Experiment with a variety of vegetables like leafy greens, zucchini, cauliflower, and bell peppers to keep your meals exciting and diverse.

Tip 5: Adjust for Activity Levels

On days when you're more physically active, it's okay to increase your calories slightly, especially from healthy carbs and protein, to replenish the energy burned during your workout. On rest days or days when you're less active, scale back on carbs and focus more on protein and fats to promote fat burning.

Tip 6: Be Patient and Consistent

Weight loss and energy gains don't happen overnight. Stay consistent with your calorie cycling plan, monitor your progress, and make small adjustments as needed. If you hit a plateau or feel your energy dipping, don't be discouraged—small tweaks to your meal plan or macronutrient balance can make a big difference.

—Creating your Metabolic Confusion meal plan involves determining your high- and low-calorie days, balancing your macronutrients, and focusing on whole, nutrient-dense foods. By following the tips for calorie cycling, you can ensure that your body stays in fat-burning mode while still feeling satisfied and energized. Meal planning and meal prepping will help you stay on track, making it easier to stick to your goals and enjoy the process along the way.

Portion Control and Tracking

Portion control and tracking are essential skills when it comes to Metabolic Confusion. While calorie cycling helps you regulate your calorie intake, proper portion control ensures that you're getting the right amounts of food without overindulging. This approach not only helps with weight loss but also prevents overeating on both low- and high-calorie days.

Let's break down why portion control and tracking matter and how to make them work for you.

Why Portion Control is Important

Even if you're eating healthy, nutrient-dense foods, eating too much of anything can still lead to overeating and interfere with your goals. Portion control is about balancing the right amount of food at each meal to make sure you're meeting your calorie and macronutrient goals without going overboard.

- **Regulates Caloric Intake**: Portion control helps you stick to your high-calorie or low-calorie day plan. Without portion control, it's easy to consume more calories than intended, even from healthy foods.
- **Prevents Mindless Eating**: When meals are prepared and portioned ahead of time, you avoid the risk of mindlessly reaching for seconds or extra snacks. Knowing how much food you're eating helps you stay aware of your intake.
- **Promotes Balanced Nutrient Distribution**: When you manage your portions, you're more likely to keep your macronutrient breakdown on track. It helps you stay within the appropriate range for protein, carbs, and fats.

How to Practice Portion Control

- **Use a Food Scale or Measuring Cups**: One of the most reliable ways to practice portion control is by using a food scale or measuring cups to weigh or measure out your food. This ensures accuracy, especially for items like meat, grains, and nuts, which can be easy to overestimate.

- **Control Serving Sizes**: Familiarize yourself with typical serving sizes for various foods. For example, a serving of protein might be around 3-4 ounces, a serving of carbs could be ½ cup cooked rice, and a serving of fats might be 1 tablespoon of olive oil or nut butter.
- **Eat Smaller, Frequent Meals**: Instead of large, heavy meals, aim for 3 balanced meals and 1-2 snacks per day. This keeps your metabolism active, prevents overeating, and helps maintain steady energy levels.

Tracking Your Food

Tracking your food intake is an effective way to stay on top of your calorie cycling plan, ensuring that you're meeting your goals for both high-calorie and low-calorie days. While it might seem like extra work at first, food tracking helps you become more mindful of what you're eating, which can be incredibly motivating.

- **Track Calories**: Use an app or journal to log everything you eat and drink. There are many apps available that allow you to scan barcodes or input foods easily, providing an accurate breakdown of your calories and macronutrients.
- **Record Macronutrient Breakdown**: Along with tracking total calories, also track the macronutrient breakdown (protein, carbs, fats). This will ensure that you're hitting the right balance for each day, which is especially important when you're following a Metabolic Confusion plan.
- **Monitor Progress**: Tracking not only helps you stay on track with your eating, but it also allows you to review your progress over time. If something isn't working, you can adjust your portions, food choices, or meal timing accordingly.

Practical Tip: Use a Simple Journal or App

Whether you use a smartphone app or a handwritten food journal, documenting your meals can help you stay consistent. Record your portion sizes, the foods you eat, and how you feel afterward—this will help you fine-tune your plan and ensure you're staying on track with your calorie cycling.

Whole Foods

When it comes to meal planning for Metabolic Confusion, focusing on whole foods is one of the best things you can do for your body. Whole foods are minimally processed and packed with the nutrients your body needs to stay healthy, support fat loss, and maintain high energy levels. By filling your diet with nutrient-dense, whole foods, you can maximize the effectiveness of your calorie cycling plan.

Why Whole Foods Matter

- **Nutrient Density**: Whole foods, like fruits, vegetables, lean proteins, and whole grains, are packed with vitamins, minerals, antioxidants, and fiber that support overall health and well-being. These foods nourish your body and provide the fuel it needs to maintain a healthy metabolism.
- **Support Metabolic Health**: Eating a variety of whole, nutrient-dense foods helps regulate blood sugar levels, balance hormones, and support a strong, active metabolism—all of which are crucial for weight loss and energy.
- **Increased Satiety**: Whole foods, especially those high in fiber, keep you feeling fuller for longer. This helps you avoid overeating and keeps hunger at bay, especially on low-calorie days when you're trying to create a deficit.

How to Focus on Whole Foods

Here's how to ensure your meals are full of whole, nutrient-dense options:

- **Fill Half Your Plate with Vegetables**: Vegetables are naturally low in calories but high in nutrients. Fill half of your plate with vegetables at each meal to increase fiber intake, promote fullness, and support digestion.
- **Choose Lean, High-Quality Proteins**: Opt for lean protein sources such as chicken, fish, turkey, and plant-based proteins like lentils and tofu. These will provide the building blocks for muscle maintenance and fat burning without excess calories.

- **Incorporate Healthy Fats**: Healthy fats from sources like avocados, nuts, seeds, and olive oil are essential for hormone balance and energy production. These fats also keep you satisfied between meals, preventing cravings and hunger.
- **Opt for Complex Carbs**: Complex carbohydrates such as quinoa, brown rice, oats, and sweet potatoes provide long-lasting energy without spiking blood sugar. They're rich in fiber, which supports digestion and helps you feel full.
- **Avoid Processed Foods**: Processed foods, which often contain added sugars, unhealthy fats, and refined carbs, can slow down your metabolism, cause energy crashes, and make it harder to lose weight. Stick to whole foods that are as close to their natural state as possible.

Simple Whole Food Meal Examples:

- Breakfast: Scrambled eggs with spinach, tomatoes, and avocado, served with a side of whole-grain toast.
- **Lunch**: Grilled chicken salad with mixed greens, cucumbers, olive oil, and lemon dressing.
- **Dinner**: Baked salmon with roasted sweet potatoes and steamed broccoli.
- **Snack**: A handful of almonds and a small apple.

Tips for Shopping and Cooking Whole Foods

- **Shop the Perimeter**: When you go to the grocery store, focus on shopping the outer aisles. This is where you'll find fresh produce, meats, and dairy (if you consume them). Avoid the inner aisles, which are typically stocked with processed foods.
- **Batch Cook**: Preparing large portions of whole foods at the beginning of the week can save time and make sticking to your meal plan easier. Roast a large batch of vegetables, cook quinoa or rice, and portion out your proteins for quick meals throughout the week.

Portion control and tracking are vital for staying on top of your Metabolic Confusion plan, helping you keep your calorie intake in check while ensuring you're getting the right balance of macronutrients. By measuring your food, tracking your meals, and adjusting your portions as needed, you'll set yourself up for success.

Part III: Tailored Meal Plans

In this section, we'll provide tailored meal plans that align with the Metabolic Confusion Diet and guide you through each phase of the journey. These meal plans will help you build the foundation for sustainable weight loss, increased energy, and a balanced approach to nutrition.

—We'll start with Week 1: Low-Carb Kickstart, which is designed to initiate fat burning, and then move on to Week 2: Protein + Moderate Carbs, to further support muscle building and metabolism activation. Each meal plan is created with endomorphs in mind, ensuring that it's effective for your unique body type while keeping your meals delicious and easy to follow.

Week 1: Low-Carb Kickstart

Week 1 is all about jump-starting your metabolism and getting your body into fat-burning mode. Since endomorphs tend to store fat more easily, a low-carb approach during this first week will help your body shift from burning carbohydrates for fuel to burning fat instead. This helps boost metabolism and set the stage for fat loss.

—On low-carb days, you'll focus on lean proteins, healthy fats, and non-starchy vegetables. You'll minimize your intake of carbohydrates, especially refined carbs like bread, pasta, and sugary foods. Instead, we'll emphasize healthy fats and protein, which will keep you feeling full and satisfied while keeping your metabolism active.

Daily Overview for Week 1

- **High-Protein, Low-Carb Meals**: Your focus will be on protein-packed meals, including lean meats, fish, eggs, tofu, and legumes.
- **Healthy Fats**: Avocados, olive oil, nuts, and seeds will be included to help keep you feeling satisfied.
- **Non-Starchy Vegetables**: Leafy greens, broccoli, zucchini, cauliflower, and bell peppers will provide fiber, vitamins, and minerals without the carbs.

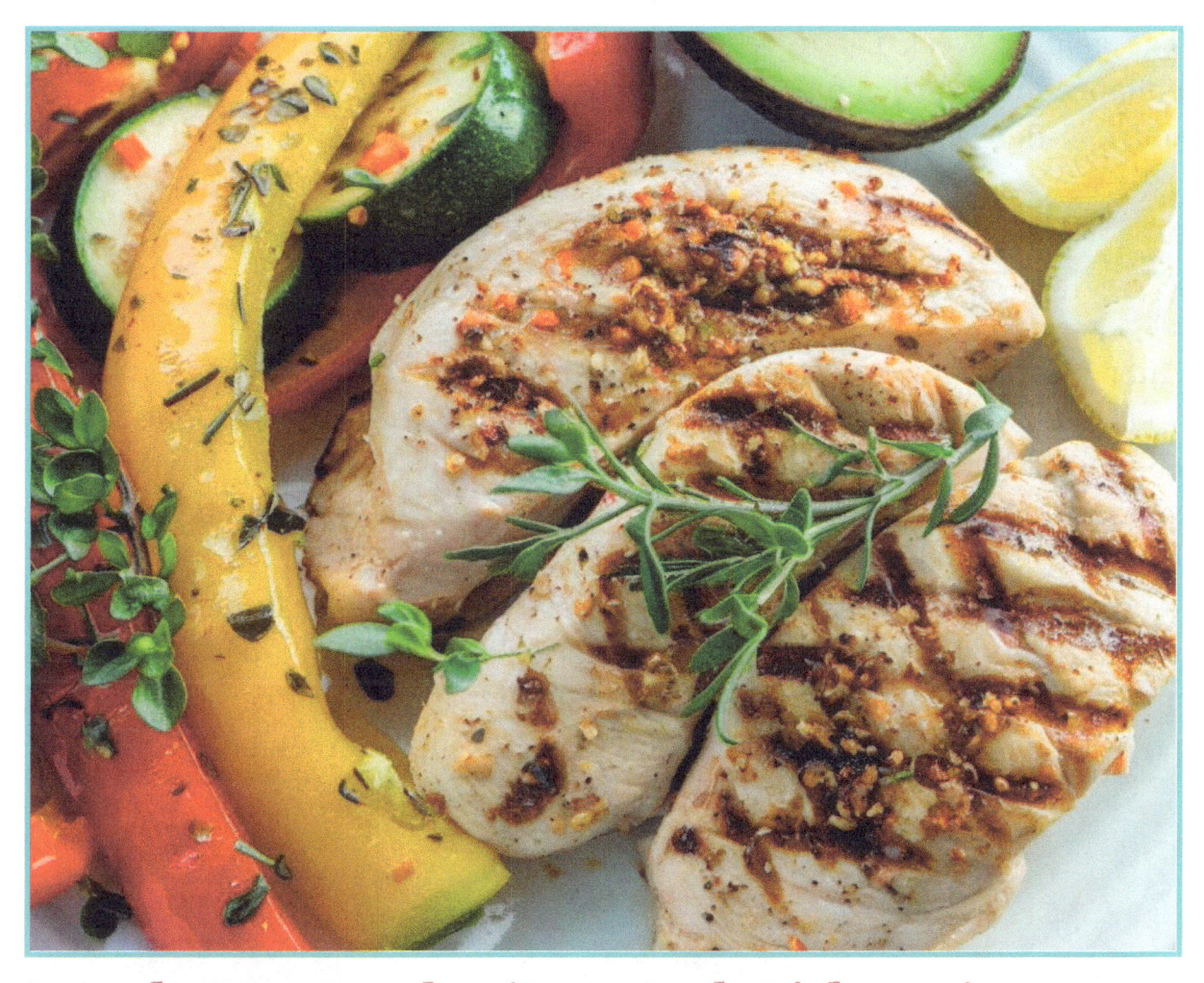

Sample Day: Week 1 (Low-Carb Kickstart)

1. **Breakfast**: Scrambled eggs with spinach and avocado, cooked in olive oil.
    a. **Tip**: Add a sprinkle of feta cheese for extra flavor and healthy fats.
2. **Snack**: A handful of almonds and a few baby carrots.
3. **Lunch**: Grilled chicken breast with a large salad (mixed greens, cucumber, tomatoes, olive oil, and lemon dressing).
4. **Snack**: A boiled egg or some Greek yogurt (unsweetened) with a few chia seeds.
5. **Dinner**: Baked salmon with steamed broccoli and roasted cauliflower.
    a. **Tip**: Add olive oil and garlic for flavor, and sprinkle with fresh herbs like parsley.

The goal of Week 1 is to reduce insulin levels, promote fat burning, and enhance metabolic function by minimizing carbs and focusing on nutrient-dense, high-protein, and healthy-fat foods.

Week 2: Protein + Moderate Carbs

After Week 1's low-carb focus, Week 2 introduces moderate carbs back into your diet, specifically complex carbohydrates that provide long-lasting energy without spiking your blood sugar. This is a perfect balance to support muscle recovery, maintain energy for workouts, and continue boosting metabolism.

—For Week 2, you'll consume moderate carbs on higher-calorie days to fuel workouts and build muscle. On low-calorie days, you'll still focus on protein and healthy fats, but you'll add in a smaller amount of carbs like sweet potatoes or quinoa to keep your energy up and support metabolic function.

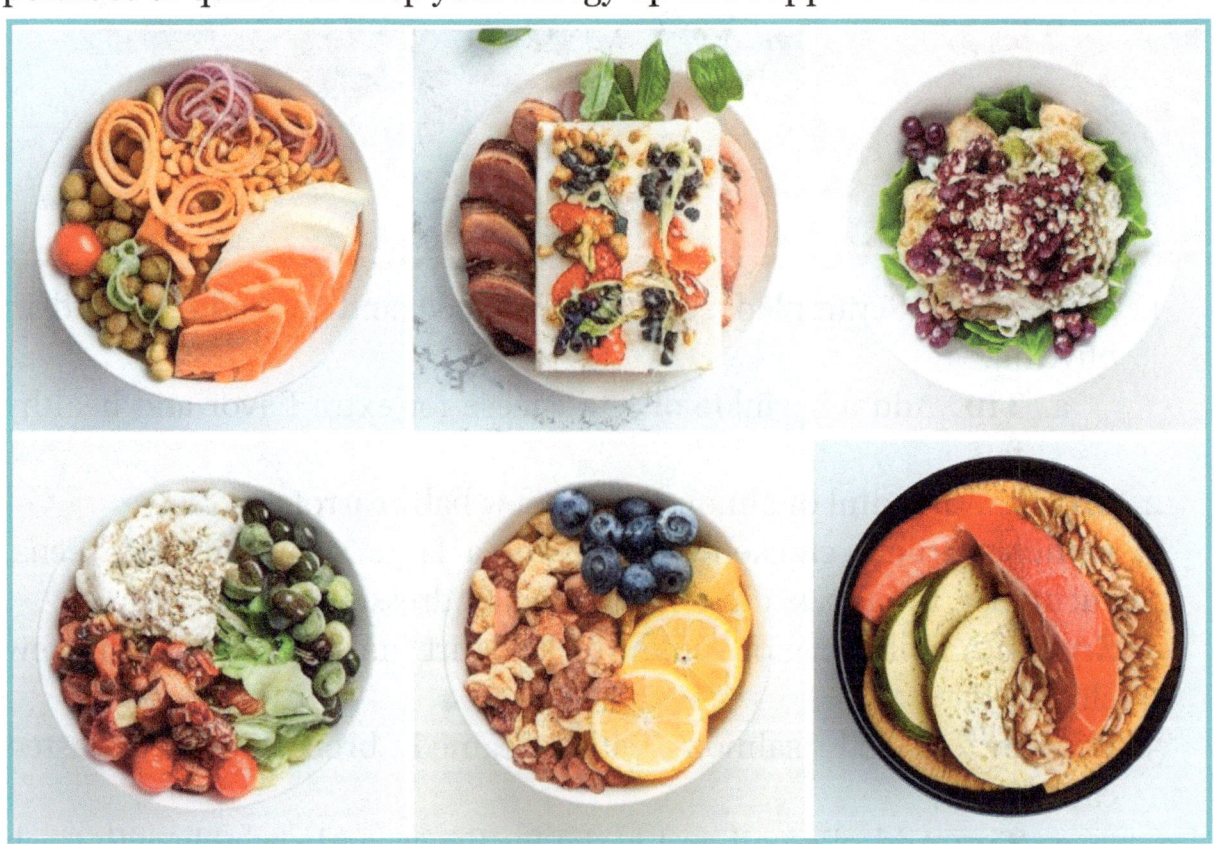

Daily Overview for Week 2

- **Protein Focus**: Continue with high-protein meals to support muscle maintenance and fat burning.
- **Moderate Carbs**: Include complex carbs such as sweet potatoes, quinoa, and whole grains in moderation to fuel your workouts.
- **Healthy Fats**: Avocados, olive oil, and nuts will still play a major role in keeping you full and satisfied.

Sample Day: Week 2 (Protein + Moderate Carbs)

1. **Breakfast**: Protein smoothie with protein powder, spinach, almond milk, and a small banana (for carbs).
    a. **Tip**: Add flaxseeds or chia seeds for extra fiber and healthy fats.
2. **Snack**: A boiled egg with a small apple.
3. **Lunch**: Turkey breast wrap with lettuce, tomatoes, avocado, and a sprinkle of olive oil, wrapped in a large lettuce leaf.
    a. **Tip**: Use hummus as a dip for added flavor and healthy fats.
4. **Snack**: Greek yogurt with a small serving of mixed berries (for a bit of natural sweetness and antioxidants).
5. **Dinner**: Grilled steak with quinoa and steamed asparagus.
    a. **Tip**: Add a drizzle of olive oil and a sprinkle of fresh lemon for a burst of flavor.

In Week 2, you'll focus on moderate carb intake that includes complex carbs to fuel your muscles and workouts while maintaining a stable metabolism. The key is to stay mindful of carb portions and balance them with lean proteins and healthy fats. This will help you continue the process of fat burning while providing sustained energy for your daily activities.

Week 3: Carb Reintroduction

Week 3 is an exciting phase in your Metabolic Confusion journey because it introduces the concept of carb reintroduction. After the initial two weeks of low-carb and moderate-carb meals, it's time to add a bit more carbohydrate into your diet. This process helps your body become more adaptable to different types of fuel while continuing to promote fat loss and boost energy.

—Carb reintroduction is designed to keep your metabolism active and ensure that your body is able to handle carbs efficiently, without going back to storing them as fat. By carefully reintroducing healthy carbs, you'll continue to keep your metabolism guessing, preventing plateaus, and avoiding the sluggishness that often accompanies long-term low-carb dieting.

Daily Overview for Week 3 (Carb Reintroduction)

- **Increased Carb Intake**: This week, you'll add healthy carbohydrates to your meals, such as whole grains, sweet potatoes, quinoa, and legumes. These carbs will fuel your workouts and help with muscle recovery.
- **Protein Focus**: Maintain your high-protein intake to ensure muscle growth and fat burning. Lean proteins will continue to be an important part of your meals.
- **Healthy Fats**: Continue incorporating healthy fats to maintain hormone balance and satiety.

Sample Day: Week 3 (Carb Reintroduction)

1. **Breakfast**: Scrambled eggs with spinach, mushrooms, and a small portion of sweet potato.
    a. **Tip**: Add a sprinkle of cheese or a drizzle of olive oil for extra healthy fats.
2. **Snack**: A handful of mixed nuts with a small serving of fruit, such as an apple or a few berries.
3. **Lunch**: Grilled chicken breast with quinoa and a mixed salad (greens, cucumber, olive oil, and balsamic vinegar).
    a. **Tip**: Add a boiled egg to the salad for more protein and healthy fats.
4. **Snack**: Greek yogurt with a tablespoon of chia seeds and a few slices of banana (this will give you natural sugars and extra fiber).
5. **Dinner**: Baked salmon with roasted sweet potato, steamed broccoli, and a drizzle of olive oil.
    a. **Tip**: Add a squeeze of lemon and fresh herbs like parsley for added flavor.

In Week 3, the goal is to start reintroducing healthy carbs in a controlled way. This allows your body to benefit from the increased energy and muscle recovery support that carbs provide while maintaining a fat-burning environment. By strategically adding carbs, you'll be able to manage your weight without sacrificing muscle or energy levels.

4, 6, and 8-Week Meal Plans

Now that you've had a taste of the tailored meal plans for Weeks 1-3, let's take a look at the bigger picture with meal plans for 4, 6, and 8 weeks. These longer-term meal plans are designed to keep your metabolism engaged, prevent plateaus, and support your goals of weight loss, muscle retention, and sustained energy.

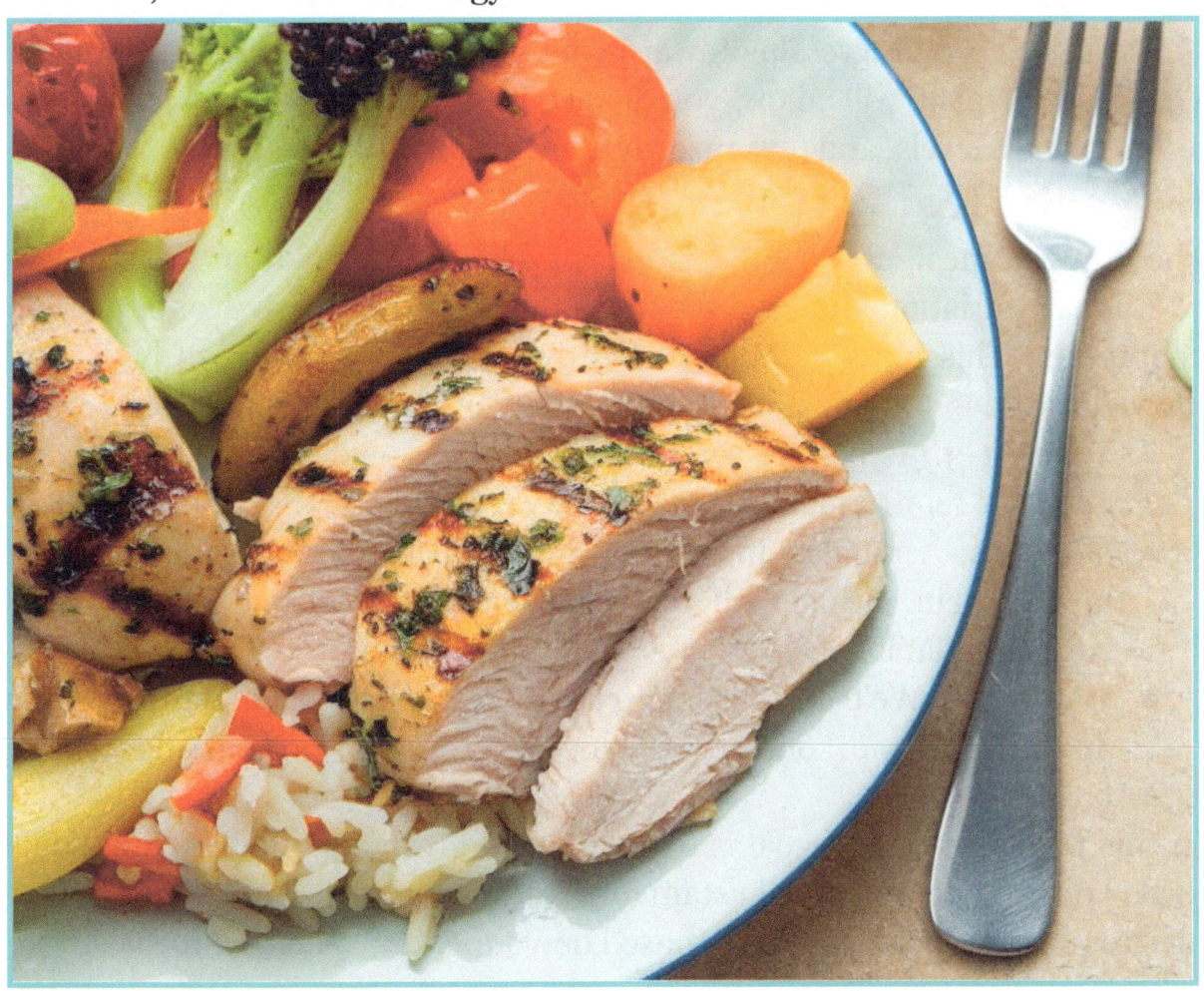

4-Week Meal Plan Overview

The 4-week meal plan combines low-carb, moderate-carb, and carb reintroduction phases, with each week designed to ramp up your metabolism, optimize fat loss, and keep things interesting. It will follow the structure we've already discussed, cycling between high-calorie days, low-calorie days, and moderate-carb days to keep your metabolism guessing.

- **Week 1:** Low-Carb Kickstart (focus on protein, healthy fats, and non-starchy vegetables)
- **Week 2:** Protein + Moderate Carbs (introducing complex carbs for energy and muscle maintenance)
- **Week 3:** Carb Reintroduction (gradually adding more carbs to fuel workouts and support metabolism)
- **Week 4:** Maintain a balance of protein, moderate carbs, and healthy fats to keep progressing toward your goals without a plateau.

This 4-week plan will allow you to get into a steady rhythm, adjust to different carb levels, and optimize your fat-burning process.

6-Week Meal Plan Overview

The 6-week meal plan builds on the previous 4 weeks and introduces additional variation to keep your metabolism responsive and prevent adaptation. This plan includes a slightly longer cycle between high- and low-calorie days and introduces more variety in carb reintroduction.

- **Week 1-3**: As before, you'll cycle between low-carb, moderate-carb, and carb reintroduction phases.
- **Week 4**: A rebalancing week where you include a combination of high-protein meals with moderate carbs for muscle recovery and continued fat loss.
- **Week 5-6**: We'll add strategic carb days to replenish muscle glycogen and increase workout performance, paired with protein and healthy fats for balance.

In this 6-week plan, the goal is to keep things fresh and challenging. You'll focus on maintaining a sustainable calorie intake, continue making progress, and adjust carb intake based on your energy needs and goals.

8-Week Meal Plan Overview

The 8-week meal plan extends the cycle even further, allowing for deep customization and longer-term progression. This plan includes strategic carb cycling and focuses on sustainable weight loss, improved energy levels, and muscle retention.

- **Week 1-3**: Follow the low-carb, moderate-carb, and carb reintroduction phases as described earlier.
- **Week 4-5**: Continue with a more flexible carb cycling approach, where you can increase carbs on high-calorie days based on activity level.
- **Week 6-7**: Begin to introduce advanced strategies like meal timing, where you'll eat larger meals earlier in the day and lighter meals in the evening. This helps with digestion and can aid in fat loss.
- **Week 8**: The final week is a maintenance phase, where you continue following the principles of carb cycling and maintain a healthy balance of protein, healthy fats, and moderate carbs. The focus is on sustainability—helping you transition to a long-term healthy eating plan that supports your lifestyle.

Sample Weekly Overview for 4, 6, and 8 Weeks

For these longer meal plans, your weekly focus will vary based on carb cycling patterns. Here's a quick breakdown:

- **High-Calorie Days (2-3 days per week):** These days will focus on moderate carbs (sweet potatoes, quinoa, etc.), protein, and healthy fats. They are scheduled around your more active or intense workout days.
- **Low-Calorie Days (2-3 days per week):** These days are lower in carbs and focus on lean proteins, vegetables, and healthy fats to promote fat loss.
- **Moderate-Carb Days (1-2 days per week):** These days will reintroduce healthy complex carbs to fuel workouts, muscle recovery, and help balance energy levels.

In Summary:

- Week 3 (Carb Reintroduction) focuses on gradually adding healthy carbs to your meals to fuel your workouts and continue supporting fat loss.
- The 4-week, 6-week, and 8-week meal plans are designed to help you progress in your journey, ensuring continued fat-burning while adjusting carbs to support your metabolism, workouts, and goals. Each week builds on the last to prevent plateaus, optimize results, and create a balanced, sustainable approach to eating.

With these meal plans in hand, you're equipped to stay on track for long-term weight loss, increased energy, and a boosted metabolism. In the next sections, we'll dive deeper into delicious recipes and tips to make these meal plans even easier to follow and enjoy!

Part IV: Recipes

Breakfasts: Energizing Options

In this section, we'll kick off with energizing breakfast options that are not only nutritious but also perfectly aligned with the Metabolic Confusion Diet. These breakfasts will set the tone for your day, fueling you with the right balance of protein, healthy fats, and complex carbs (when appropriate) to keep your metabolism active and your energy levels high. Each recipe is designed to be simple, delicious, and nourishing to help you feel your best.

Recipe 1: Avocado and Egg Scramble

A hearty, protein-packed scramble with the richness of avocado, this breakfast is designed to keep you full and satisfied until your next meal. It's perfect for a low-carb day to fuel your morning and stabilize blood sugar levels. The healthy fats from the avocado and eggs will keep you feeling energized without a sugar crash.

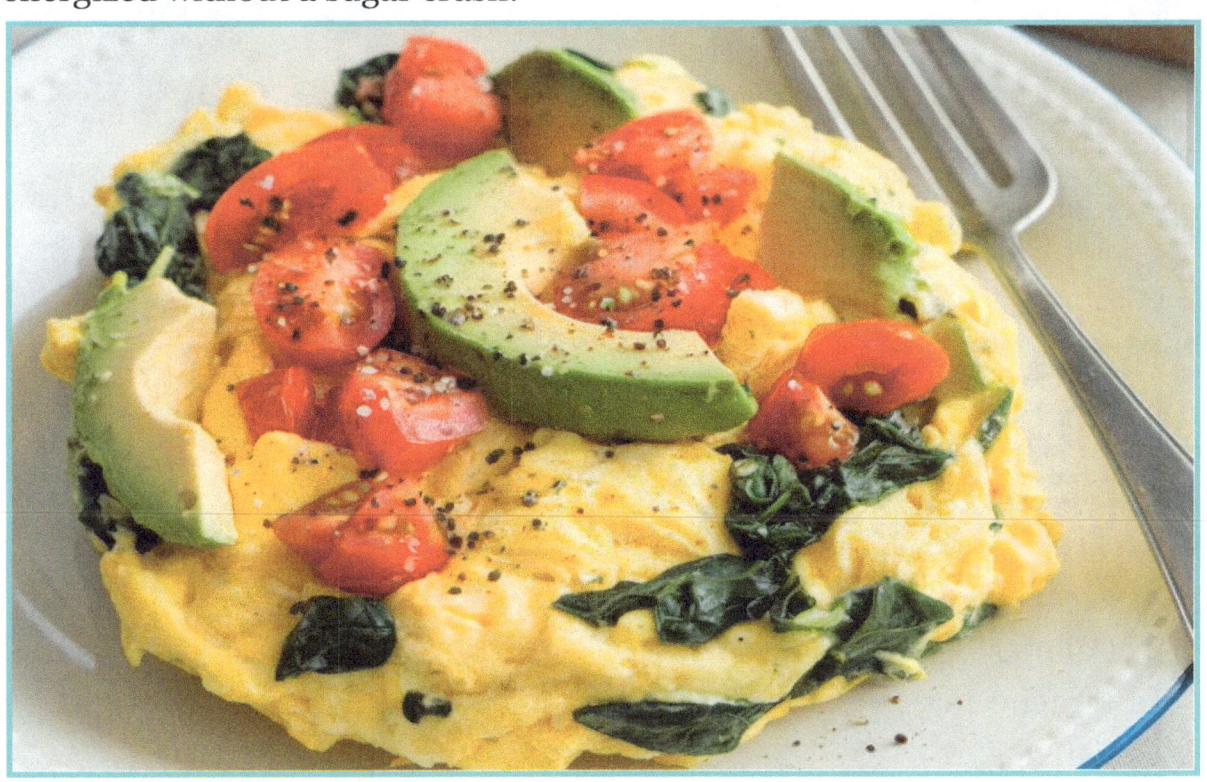

Ingredients:
- 2 large eggs
- 1/2 avocado, sliced
- 1/4 cup diced tomatoes
- 1/4 cup spinach, chopped
- 1 tablespoon olive oil
- Salt and pepper, to taste

Instructions:
1. Heat olive oil in a non-stick skillet over medium heat.
2. Add spinach and tomatoes to the pan, sautéing for about 2 minutes until the spinach wilts.
3. Crack the eggs into the pan and scramble gently. Stir occasionally until the eggs are cooked through but still soft.
4. Remove from heat and top with sliced avocado. Season with salt and pepper to taste.

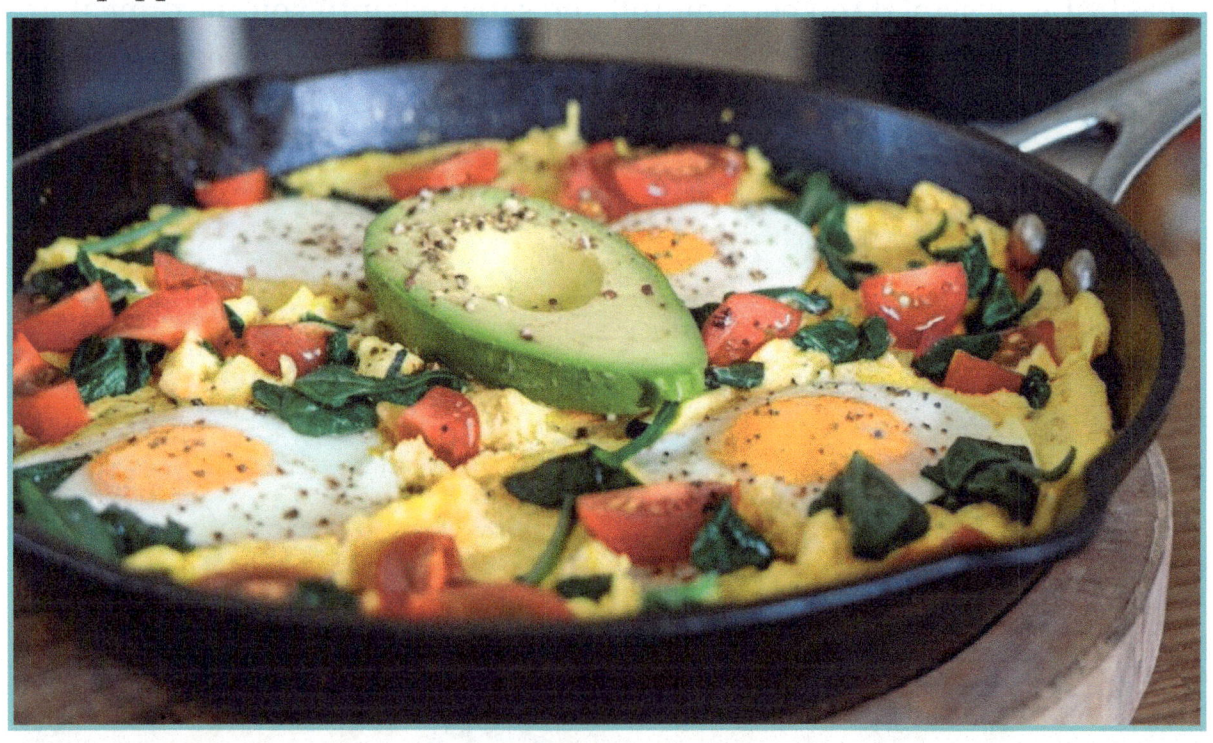

Nutrition per Serving:
- ☐ Calories: 310
- ☐ Protein: 16g
- ☐ Fat: 25g

- ☐ Carbohydrates: 8g
- ☐ Fiber: 6g

Tip: For added flavor, you can sprinkle some red pepper flakes or fresh herbs like parsley or cilantro on top.

Recipe 2: Chia Seed Pudding with Berries

A light yet satisfying breakfast, this chia seed pudding is packed with fiber, healthy fats, and antioxidants from the berries. It's perfect for a moderate-carb day where you can incorporate a bit of fruit for a natural energy boost while keeping your metabolism revved up.

Ingredients:
- 3 tablespoons chia seeds
- 1/2 cup unsweetened almond milk
- 1/4 cup Greek yogurt (unsweetened)
- 1/2 teaspoon vanilla extract
- 1/4 teaspoon cinnamon
- 1/2 cup mixed berries (blueberries, raspberries, or strawberries)

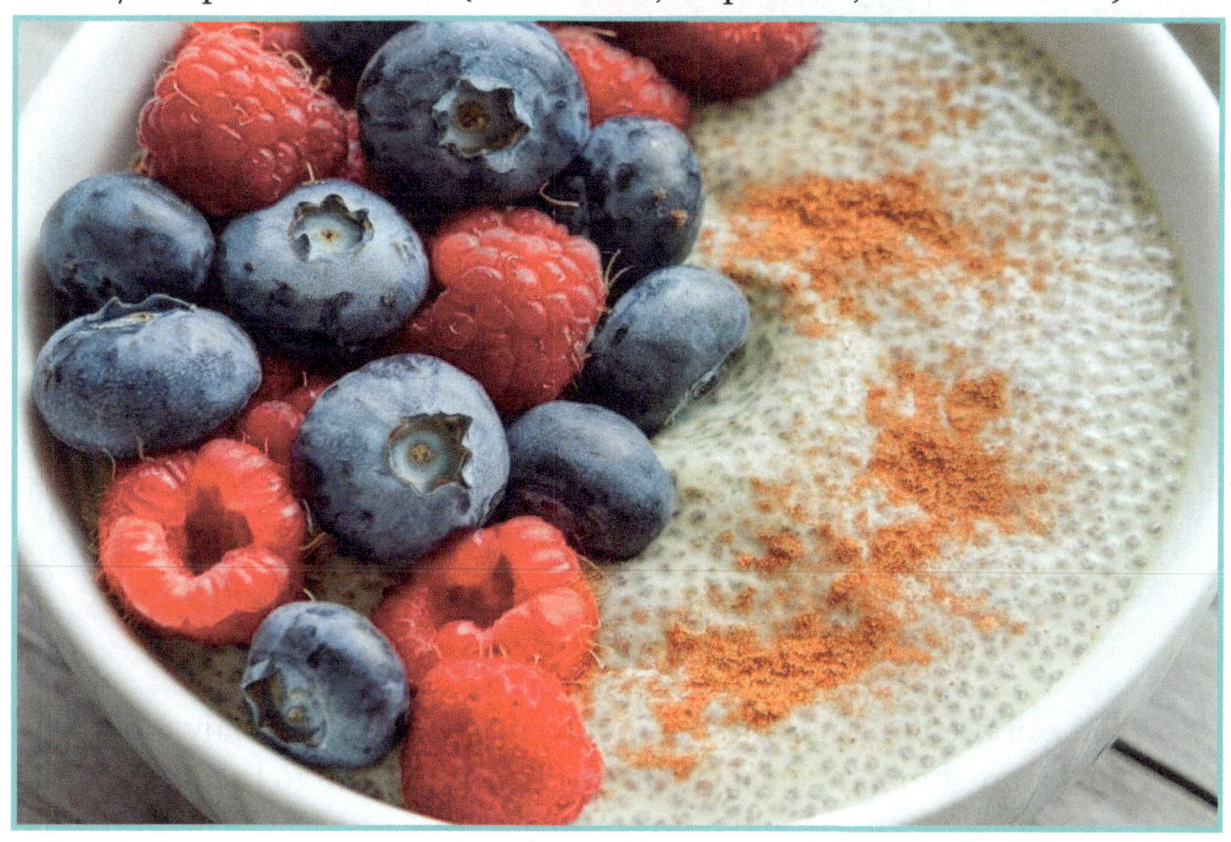

Instructions:
1. In a bowl, combine chia seeds, almond milk, Greek yogurt, vanilla extract, and cinnamon.
2. Stir well, then cover and refrigerate for at least 4 hours or overnight, allowing the chia seeds to absorb the liquid and thicken.
3. Before serving, stir the pudding and top with fresh berries.

Nutrition per Serving:
- ☐ Calories: 240
- ☐ Protein: 11g
- ☐ Fat: 14g
- ☐ Carbohydrates: 19g
- ☐ Fiber: 11g

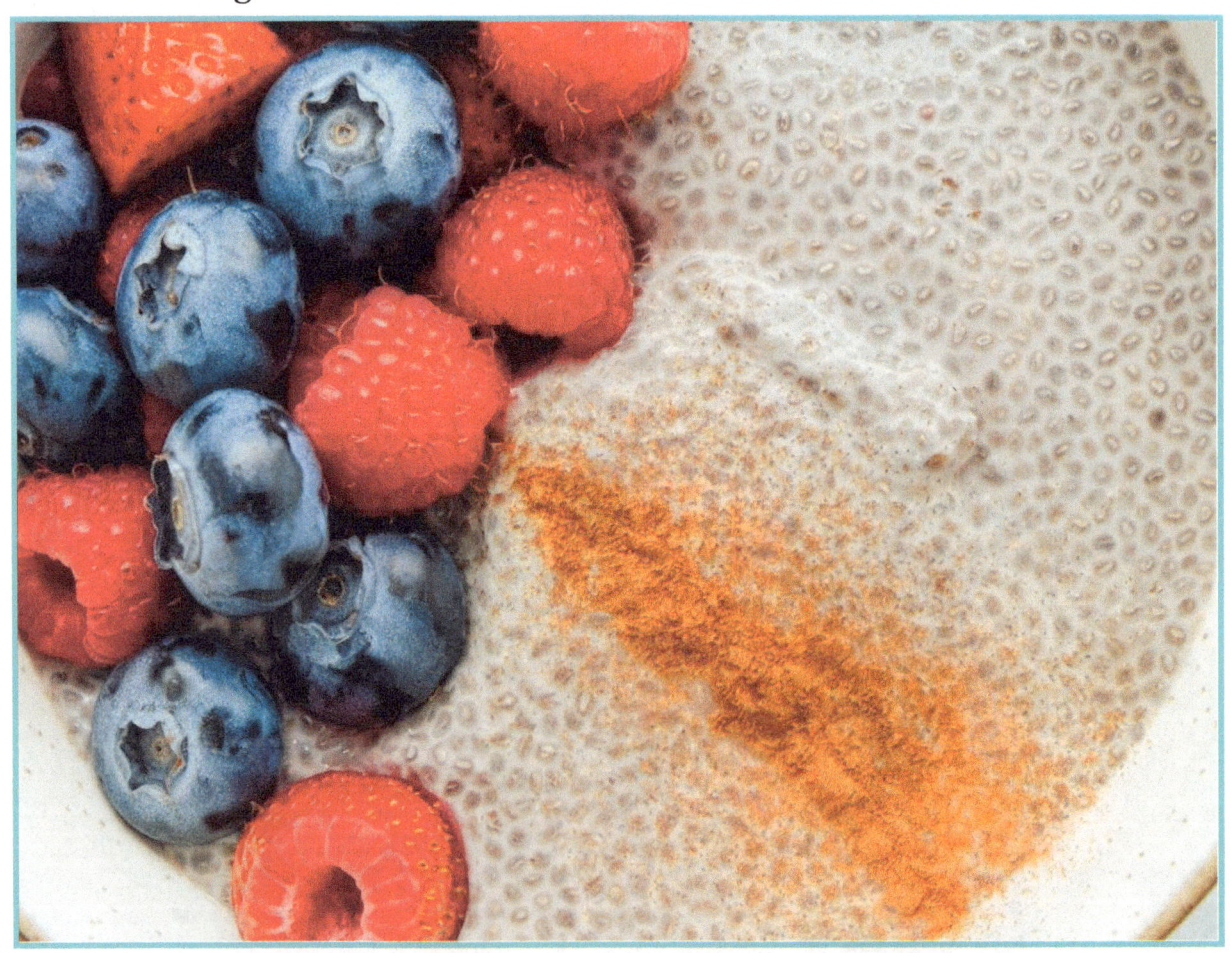

Tip: You can prepare this pudding in advance and have it ready for several days. Just store it in individual jars for an easy grab-and-go breakfast.

Recipe 3: Sweet Potato and Turkey Breakfast Bowl

This nutrient-packed breakfast bowl includes the perfect balance of lean protein, complex carbs, and healthy fats to fuel your morning. It's a great choice for a high-calorie day to support muscle repair and energy levels, especially on days when you need that extra boost.

Ingredients:
- 1 medium sweet potato, peeled and diced
- 1/2 cup cooked ground turkey (lean)
- 1/4 avocado, sliced
- 1 tablespoon olive oil
- 1/4 teaspoon smoked paprika
- Salt and pepper, to taste
- Fresh cilantro or parsley for garnish (optional)

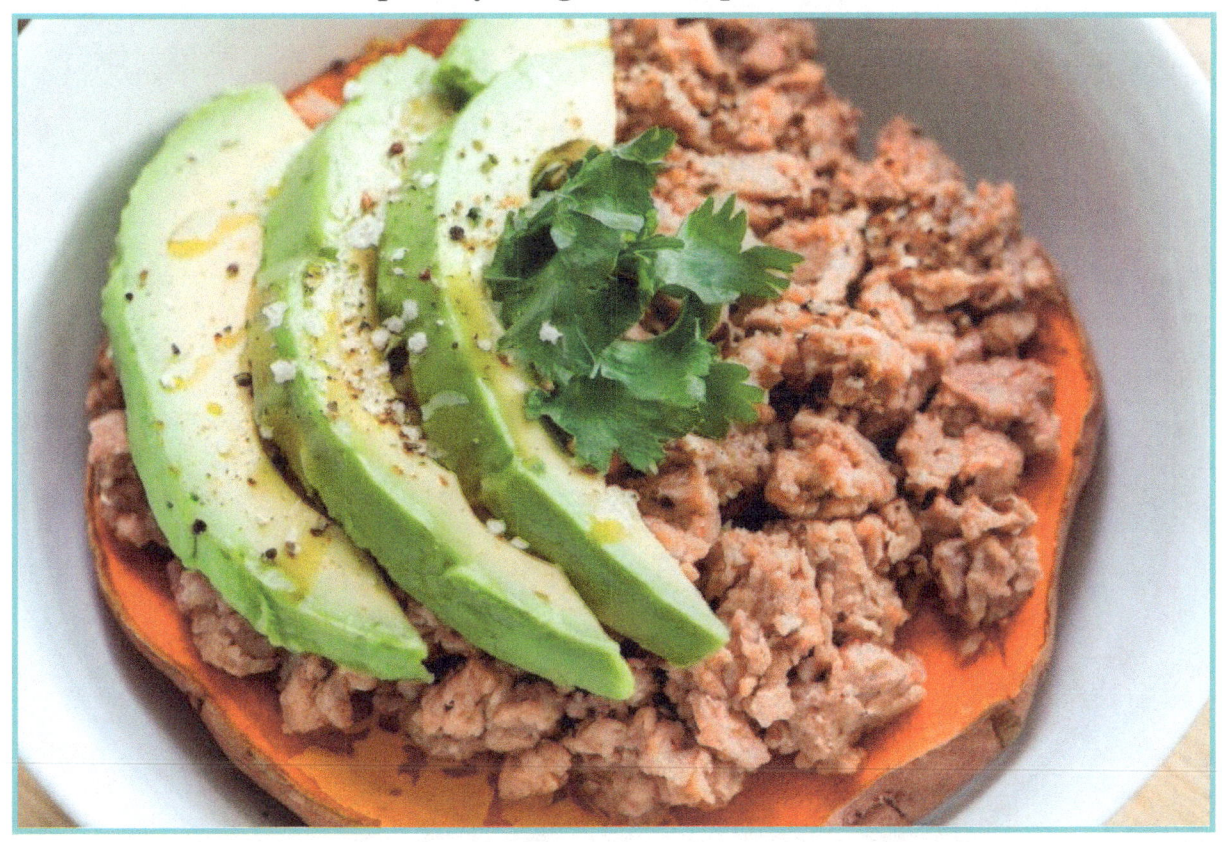

Instructions:
1. Heat olive oil in a skillet over medium heat. Add the diced sweet potato and sauté for about 8-10 minutes, or until softened and lightly browned. Season with smoked paprika, salt, and pepper.

2. In a separate pan, cook the ground turkey over medium heat until browned and cooked through (about 5-7 minutes).
3. Assemble the bowl by layering the sautéed sweet potatoes, cooked turkey, and sliced avocado. Garnish with fresh cilantro or parsley for added flavor.

Nutrition per Serving:
- ☐ Calories: 380
- ☐ Protein: 28g
- ☐ Fat: 24g
- ☐ Carbohydrates: 24g
- ☐ Fiber: 7g

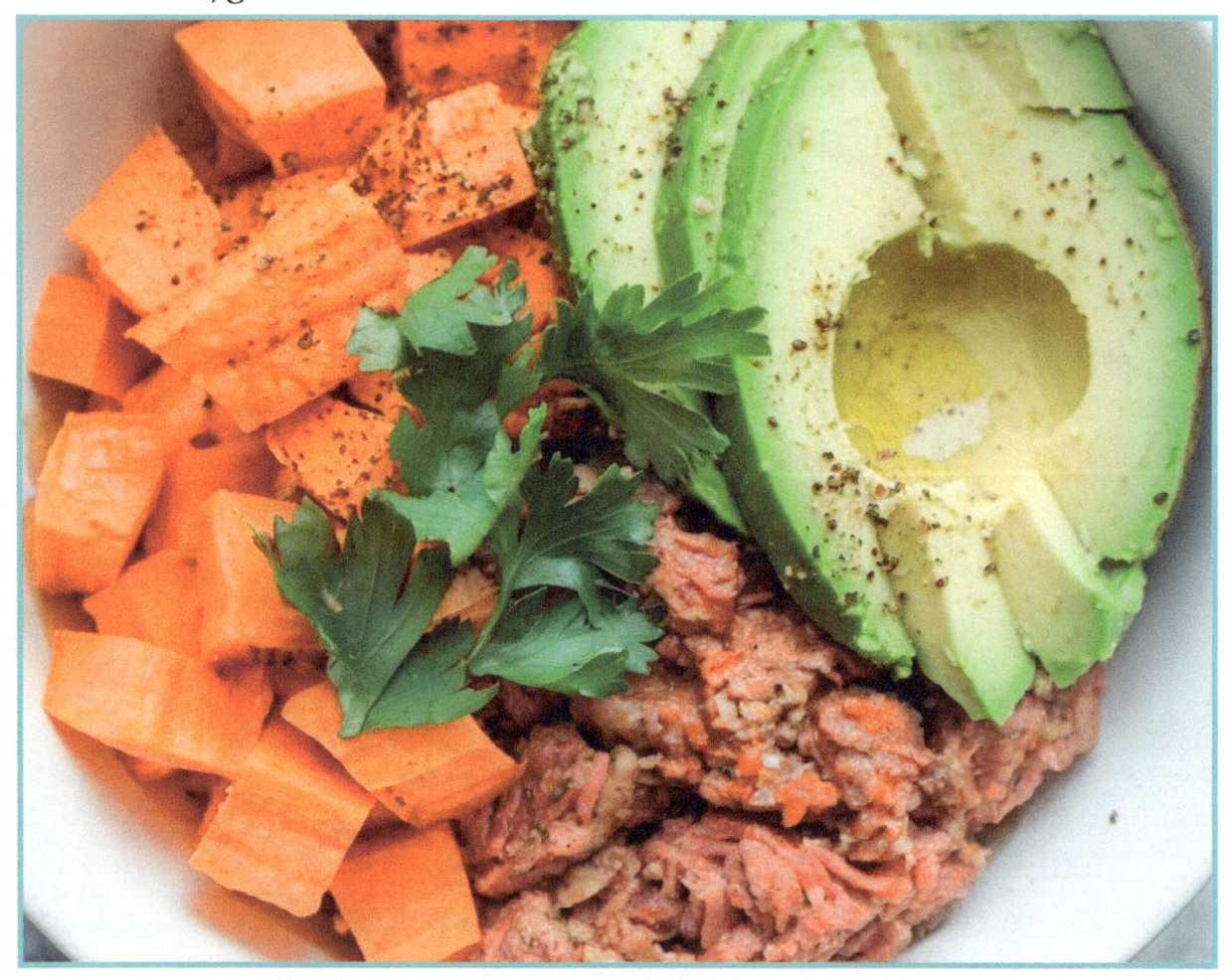

Tip: You can make this breakfast even easier by meal prepping the sweet potatoes and ground turkey ahead of time, so your mornings are quick and hassle-free.

Lunches: Satisfying Meals

Lunch is an essential meal to keep your energy levels up throughout the day. Whether it's a low-calorie day or a moderate-carb day, these lunch options are packed with protein, healthy fats, and vegetables, ensuring that you stay satisfied and fueled without overloading on calories. Let's get started!

Recipe 1: Grilled Chicken Salad with Avocado and Tahini Dressing

This vibrant salad is a delicious protein-packed lunch with the healthy fats from avocado and the rich, creamy tahini dressing. It's perfect for a moderate-carb day when you want a balanced meal that keeps you full and satisfied. The chicken provides lean protein, and the vegetables offer a variety of essential vitamins and minerals.

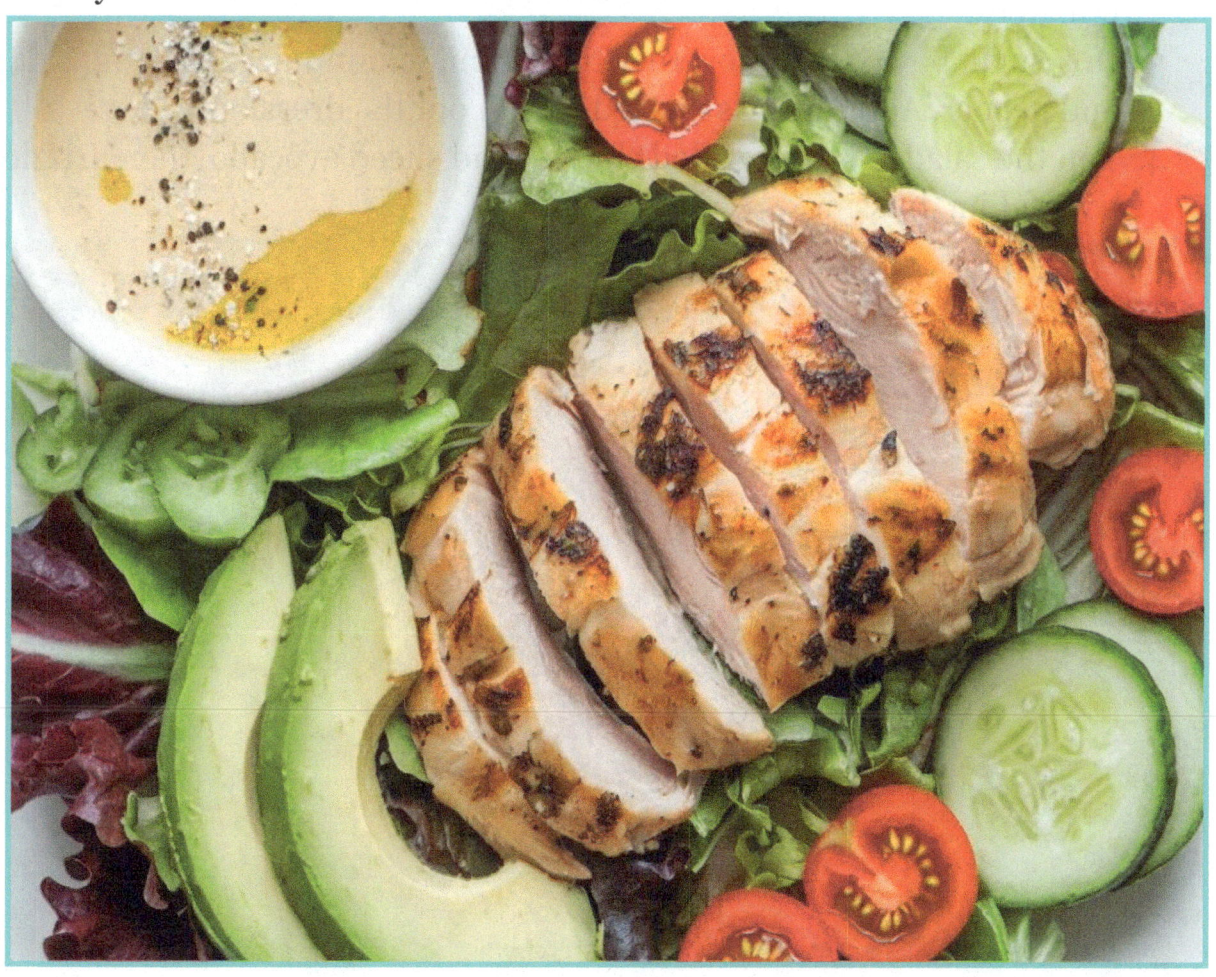

54

Ingredients:
- 4 oz grilled chicken breast, sliced
- 1/2 avocado, sliced
- 2 cups mixed greens (spinach, kale, arugula)
- 1/4 cup cucumber, sliced
- 1/4 cup cherry tomatoes, halved
- 1 tablespoon tahini
- 1 tablespoon lemon juice
- 1 teaspoon olive oil
- Salt and pepper, to taste

Instructions:
1. Grill the chicken breast on medium heat until cooked through (about 5-7 minutes per side), then slice into strips.
2. In a large bowl, combine the mixed greens, cucumber, and cherry tomatoes.
3. In a small bowl, whisk together the tahini, lemon juice, olive oil, salt, and pepper. Add water as needed to thin out the dressing.
4. Top the salad with the grilled chicken and sliced avocado, then drizzle with tahini dressing.

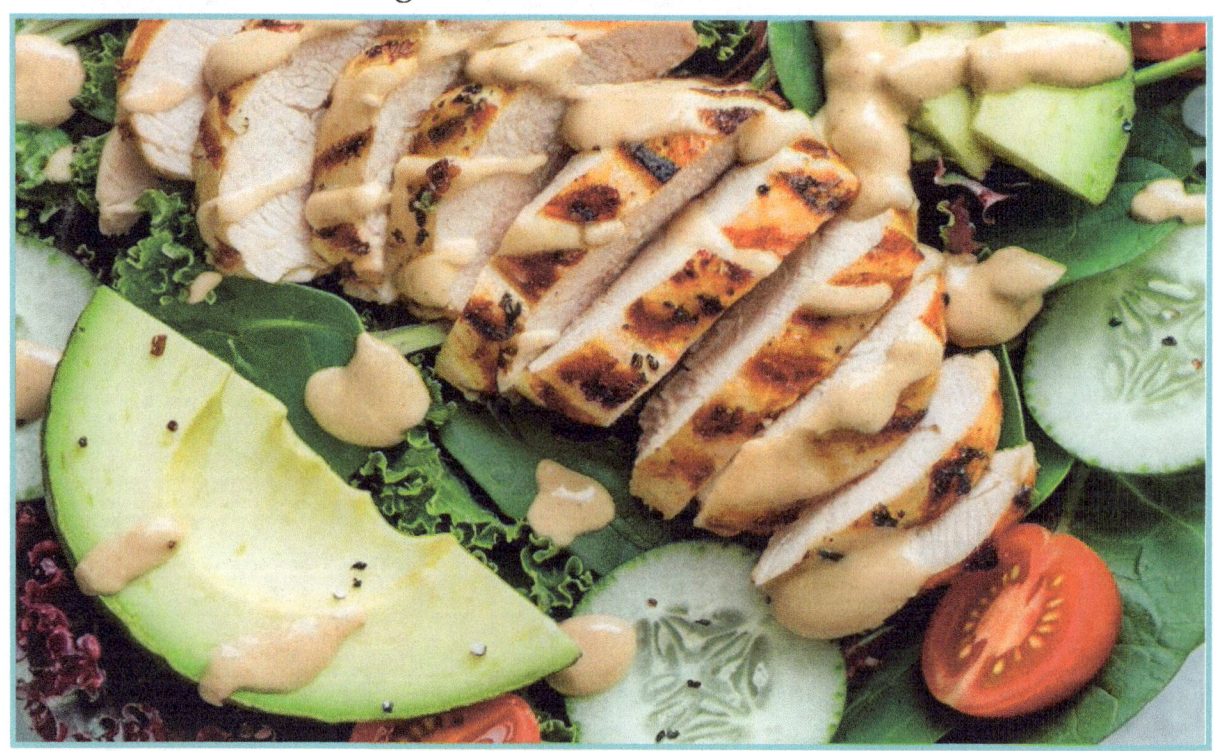

Nutrition per Serving:
- ☐ Calories: 380
- ☐ Protein: 30g
- ☐ Fat: 25g
- ☐ Carbohydrates: 13g
- ☐ Fiber: 9g

Tip: For added texture, sprinkle some sunflower seeds or chopped nuts on top!

Recipe 2: Turkey Lettuce Wraps with Avocado and Hummus

These refreshing and light lettuce wraps are a perfect low-calorie lunch option, with lean turkey, creamy avocado, and a scoop of hummus for flavor. They're easy to prepare and keep you feeling satisfied without the carbs. Perfect for a low-calorie day when you want something light yet filling.

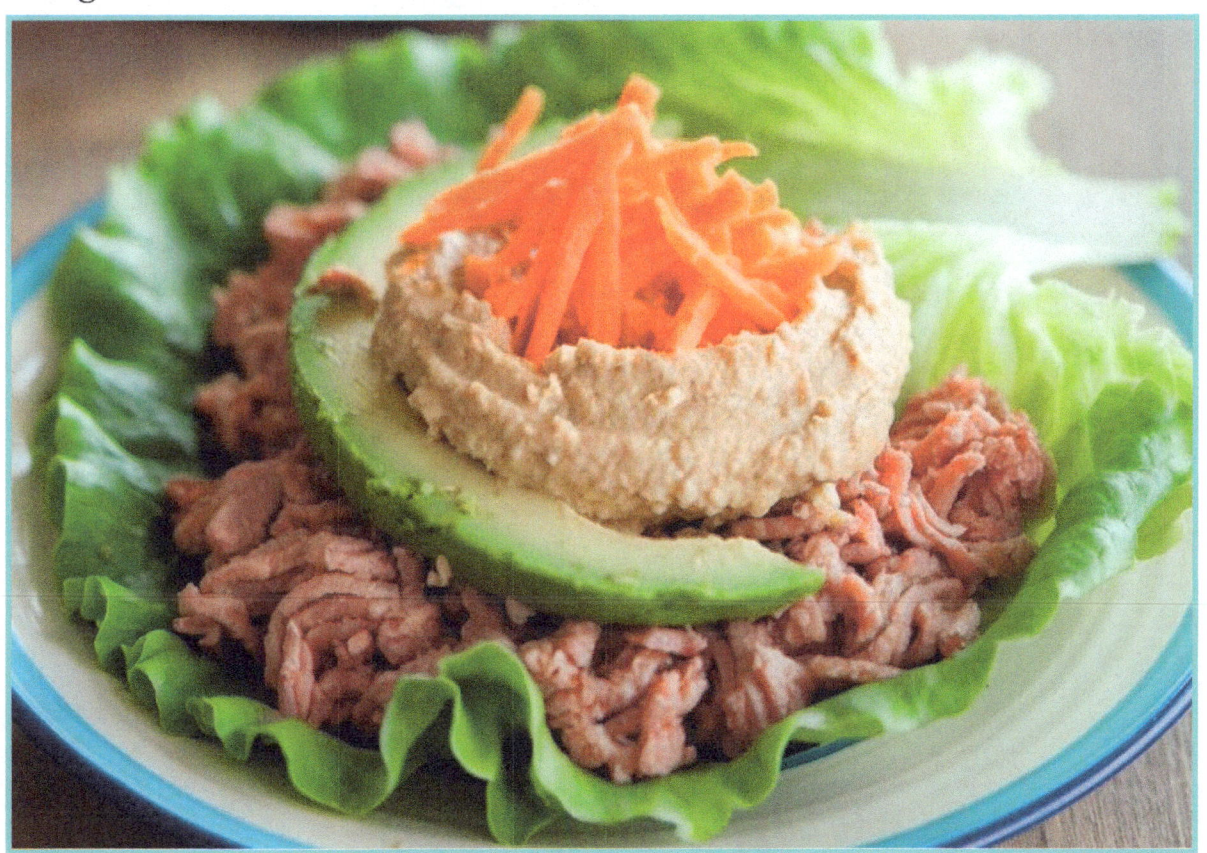

Ingredients:
- 4 oz lean ground turkey
- 1/4 teaspoon garlic powder
- 1 tablespoon olive oil
- 2 large romaine lettuce leaves
- 1/4 avocado, sliced
- 2 tablespoons hummus
- 1/4 cup shredded carrots
- Salt and pepper, to taste

Instructions:
1. In a skillet, heat the olive oil over medium heat and cook the ground turkey until browned (about 7-8 minutes). Season with garlic powder, salt, and pepper.
2. Lay the romaine lettuce leaves flat on a plate.
3. Spread hummus on each lettuce leaf, then top with the cooked turkey, avocado slices, and shredded carrots.
4. Roll up the lettuce leaves into wraps and enjoy!

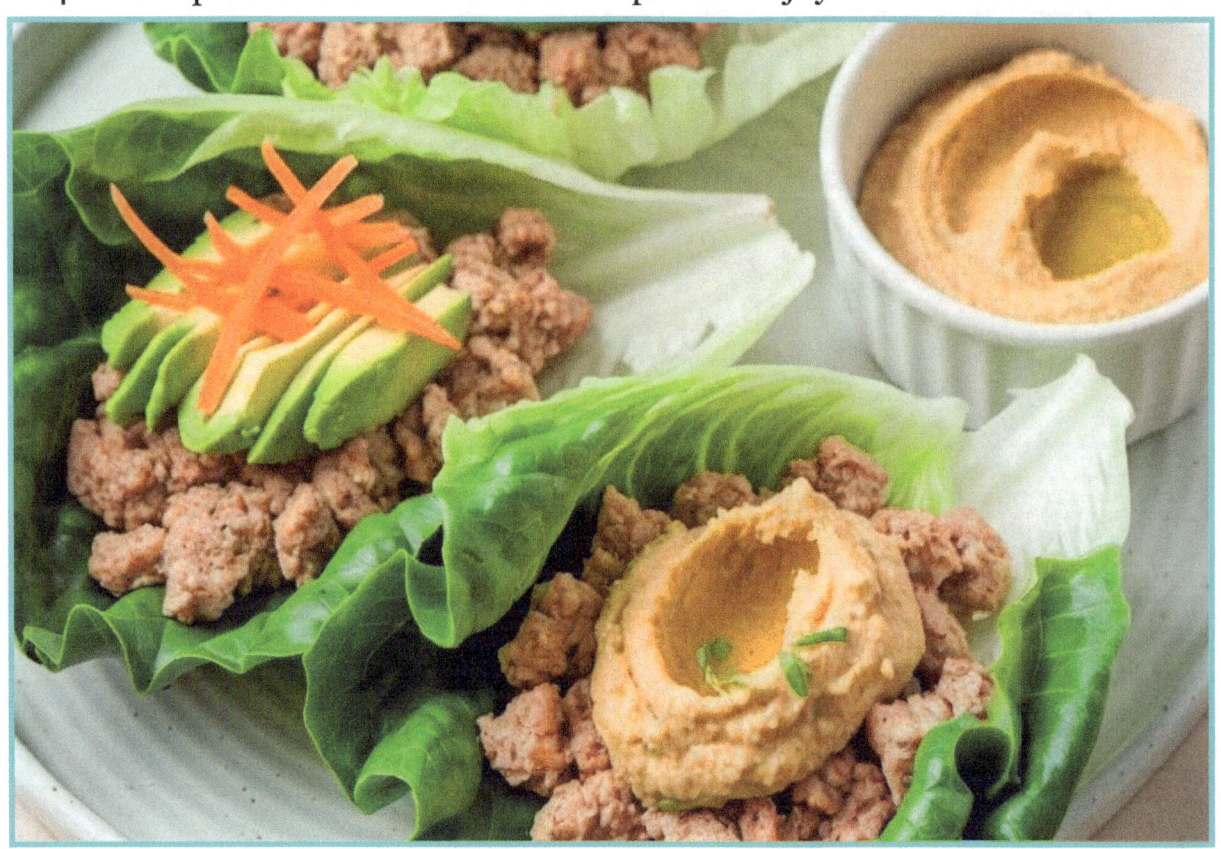

Nutrition per Serving:
- Calories: 290
- Protein: 28g
- Fat: 18g
- Carbohydrates: 10g
- Fiber: 6g

Tip: Add a sprinkle of fresh herbs, like cilantro or parsley, for extra freshness!

Recipe 3: Quinoa and Black Bean Bowl with Lime and Cilantro

A vibrant and flavorful meal that's perfect for a moderate-carb day, this quinoa and black bean bowl is packed with plant-based protein and fiber. The quinoa provides complex carbs that will fuel your energy needs, while the black beans and veggies support your metabolism.

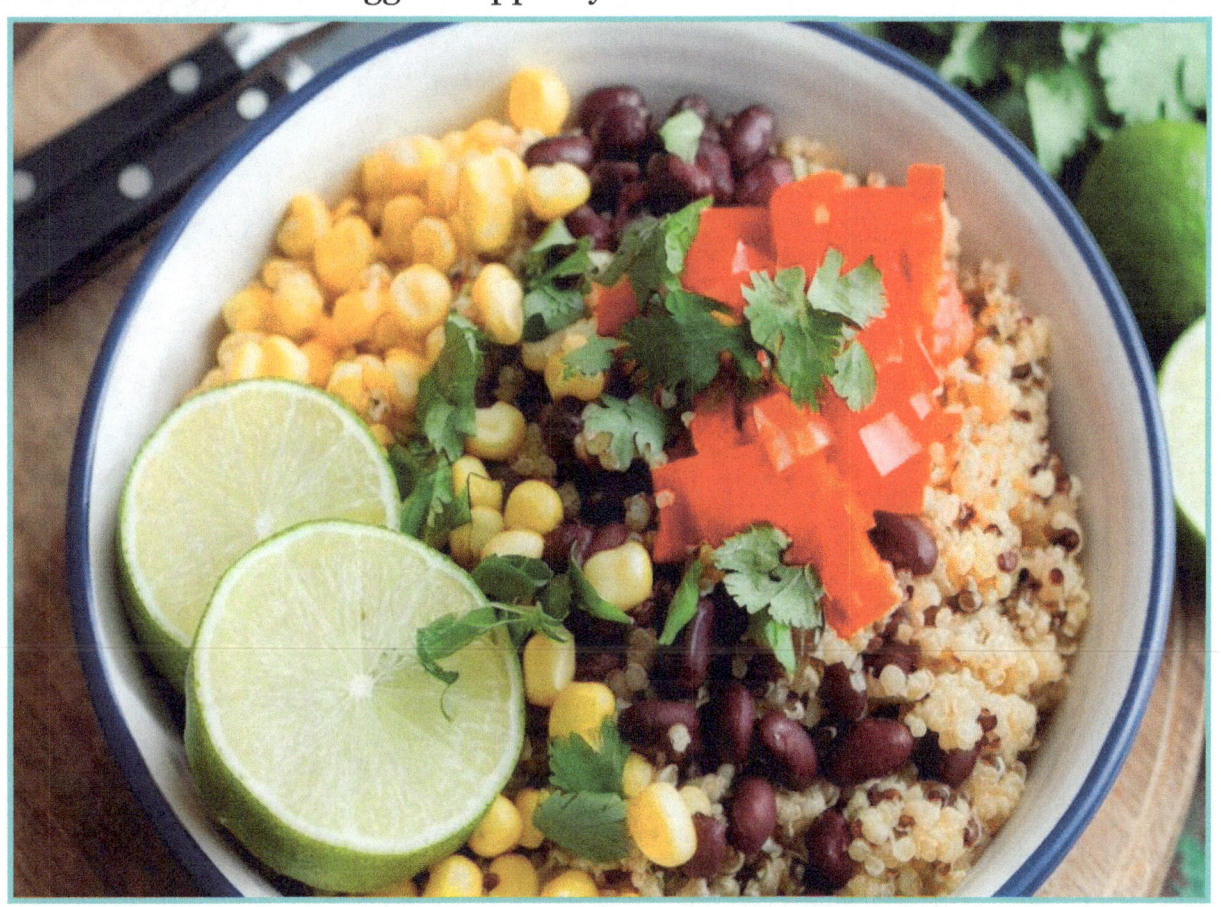

Ingredients:
- 1/2 cup cooked quinoa
- 1/2 cup black beans, drained and rinsed
- 1/4 cup corn kernels (fresh or frozen)
- 1/4 cup diced red bell pepper
- 1 tablespoon olive oil
- 1 tablespoon lime juice
- 1 tablespoon chopped cilantro
- Salt and pepper, to taste

Instructions:
1. In a skillet, heat olive oil over medium heat. Add the diced bell pepper and corn, and sauté for about 5 minutes until softened.
2. In a bowl, combine the cooked quinoa, black beans, sautéed bell pepper and corn, and lime juice.
3. Top with fresh cilantro, salt, and pepper to taste.

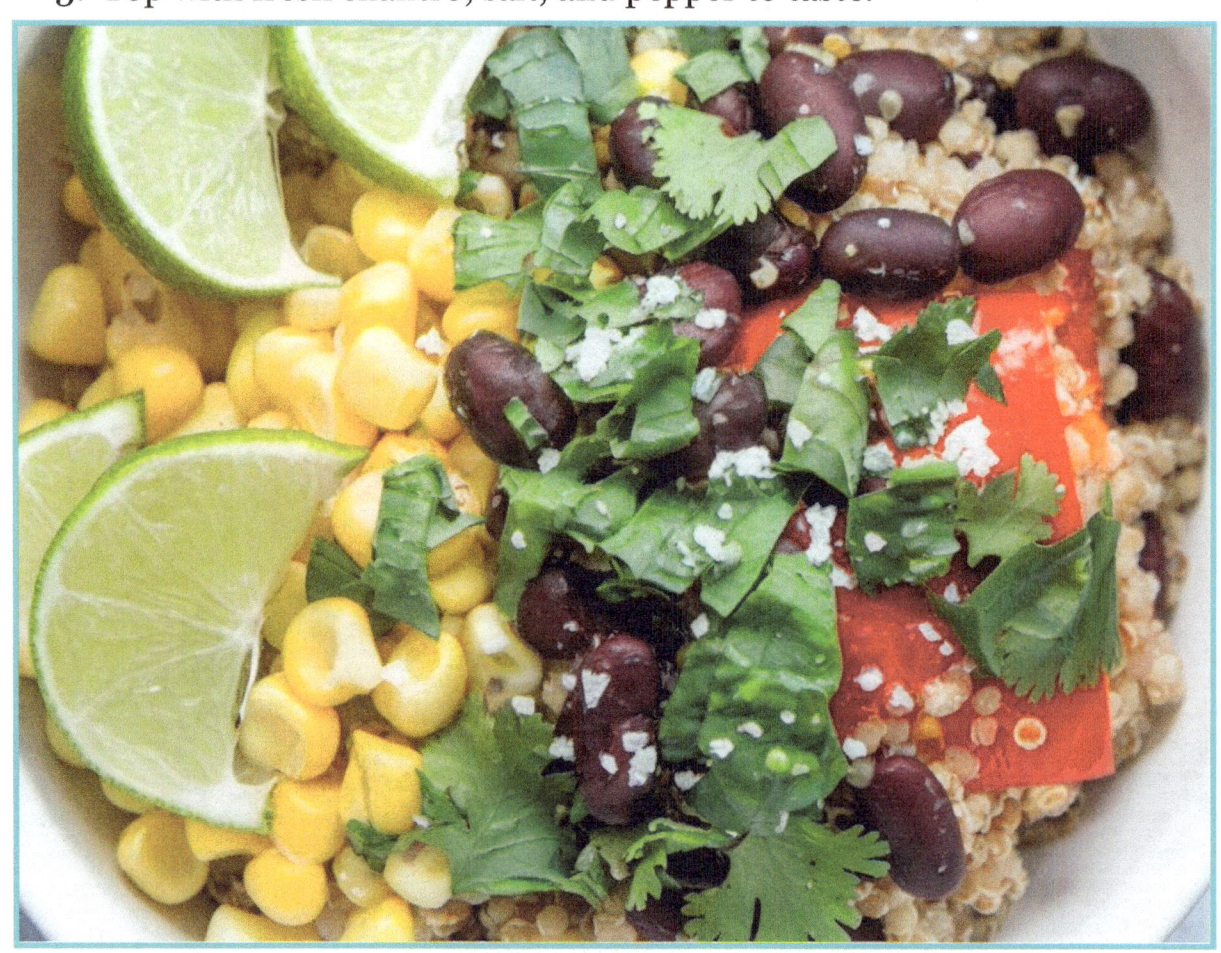

Nutrition per Serving:
- ☐ Calories: 350
- ☐ Protein: 13g
- ☐ Fat: 12g
- ☐ Carbohydrates: 45g
- ☐ Fiber: 10g

Tip: Add a dollop of Greek yogurt or avocado on top for extra creaminess!

Dinners: Low-Calorie Recipes

For dinner, we focus on keeping the meals light and satisfying while still offering enough protein to support muscle repair and healthy fat to promote satiety. These low-calorie dinner options are perfect for low-calorie days, helping you stay within your calorie goals without sacrificing flavor.

Recipe 1: Lemon Herb Baked Salmon with Steamed Asparagus

This baked salmon is an excellent source of healthy omega-3 fatty acids, and paired with steamed asparagus, it's a low-calorie dinner that's also rich in nutrients. The lemon and herbs add brightness to the meal, making it fresh and flavorful without extra calories.

Ingredients:
- 4 oz salmon fillet
- 1 tablespoon olive oil
- 1 tablespoon lemon juice
- 1/2 teaspoon dried dill
- Salt and pepper, to taste
- 1 cup asparagus, trimmed

Instructions:
1. Preheat the oven to 400°F (200°C). Place the salmon fillet on a baking sheet lined with parchment paper.

2. Drizzle olive oil and lemon juice over the salmon, then sprinkle with dill, salt, and pepper.
3. Bake for 12-15 minutes, or until the salmon is cooked through.
4. Steam the asparagus for about 5-7 minutes until tender, then season with a bit of salt and olive oil.
5. Serve the salmon with the steamed asparagus on the side.

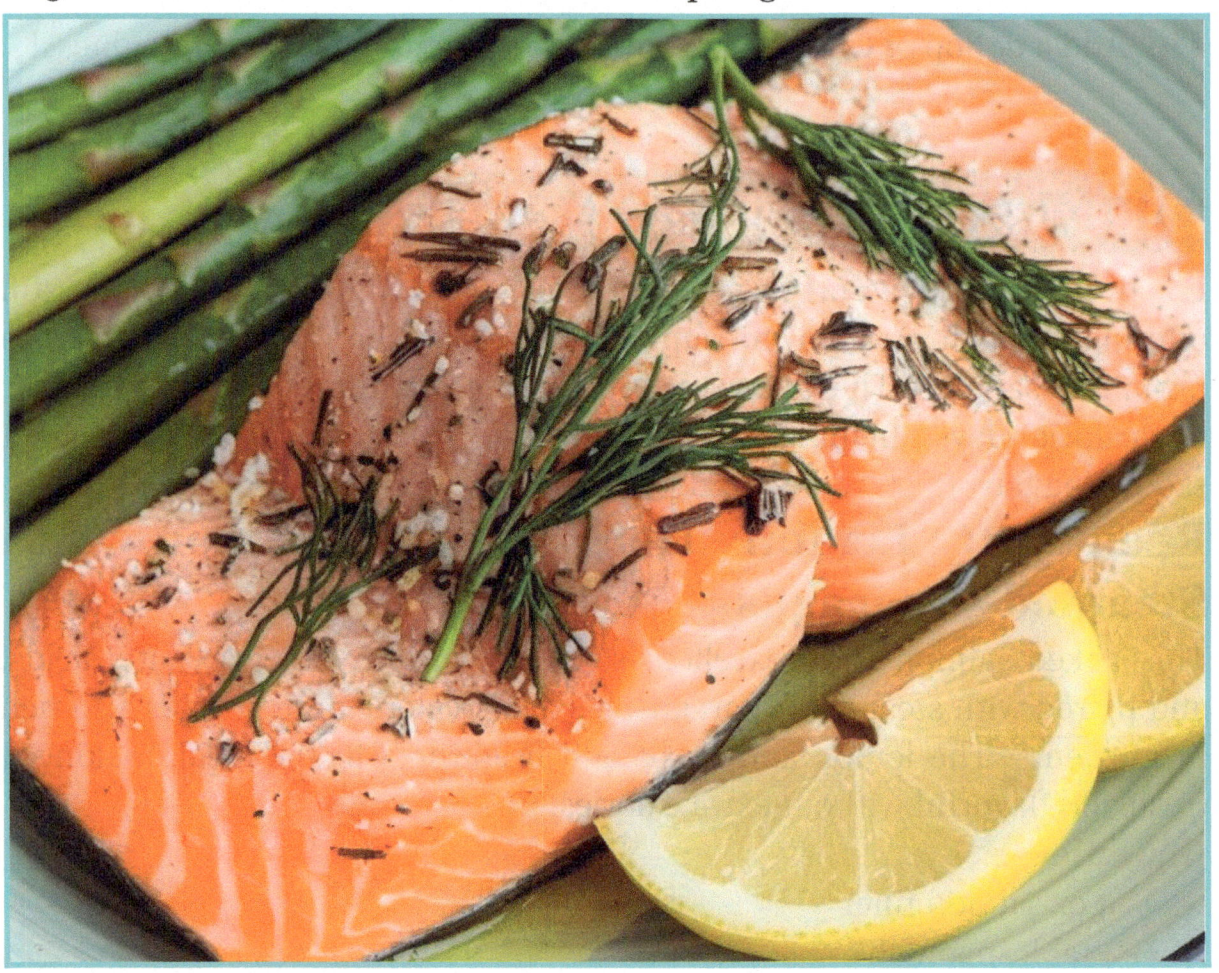

Nutrition per Serving:
- ☐ Calories: 310
- ☐ Protein: 30g
- ☐ Fat: 20g
- ☐ Carbohydrates: 7g
- ☐ Fiber: 4g

Tip: For extra flavor, top the salmon with fresh herbs like parsley or a sprinkle of garlic powder!

Recipe 2: Zucchini Noodles with Turkey Meatballs

This healthy and light version of spaghetti uses zucchini noodles as a low-calorie alternative, paired with lean turkey meatballs for protein. The meal is savory, filling, and perfect for a low-calorie day.

Ingredients:
- 2 medium zucchinis, spiralized into noodles
- 4 oz ground turkey
- 1/4 teaspoon garlic powder
- 1/4 teaspoon onion powder
- 1 tablespoon olive oil
- 1/2 cup marinara sauce (sugar-free)
- Salt and pepper, to taste

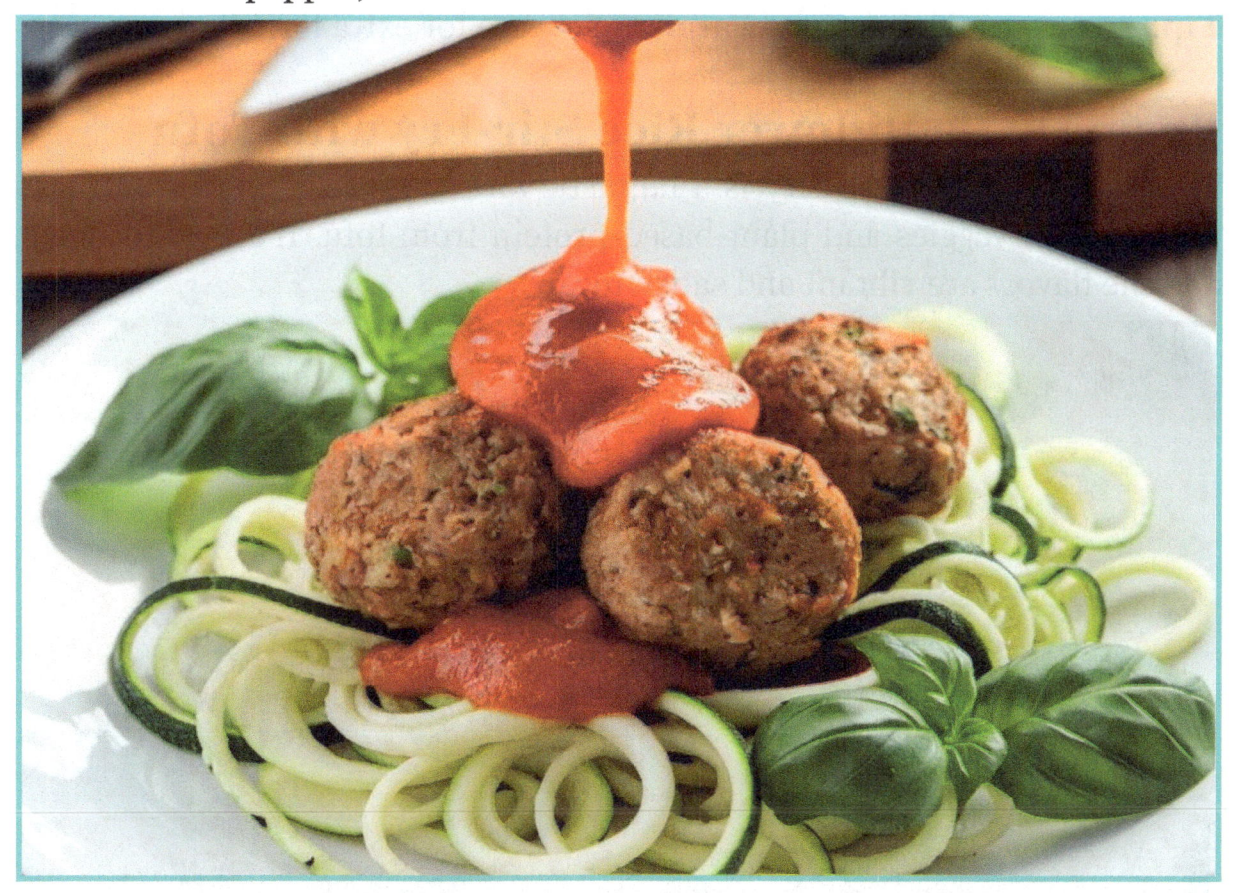

Instructions:
1. Preheat the oven to 375°F (190°C). In a bowl, combine the ground turkey, garlic powder, onion powder, salt, and pepper. Roll into small meatballs.

2. Place the meatballs on a baking sheet lined with parchment paper and bake for 12-15 minutes until fully cooked.
3. While the meatballs bake, heat olive oil in a pan over medium heat. Sauté the zucchini noodles for about 3-4 minutes until tender.
4. Once the meatballs are done, toss them in marinara sauce and serve over the zucchini noodles.

Nutrition per Serving:
- ☐ Calories: 270
- ☐ Protein: 30g
- ☐ Fat: 14g
- ☐ Carbohydrates: 12g
- ☐ Fiber: 4g

Tip: Add a sprinkle of grated Parmesan cheese for extra flavor!

Recipe 3: Cauliflower Rice Stir-Fry with Tofu

This cauliflower rice stir-fry is a fantastic low-calorie dinner option that's packed with veggies and plant-based protein from tofu. It's easy to make, and the flavors are vibrant and satisfying.

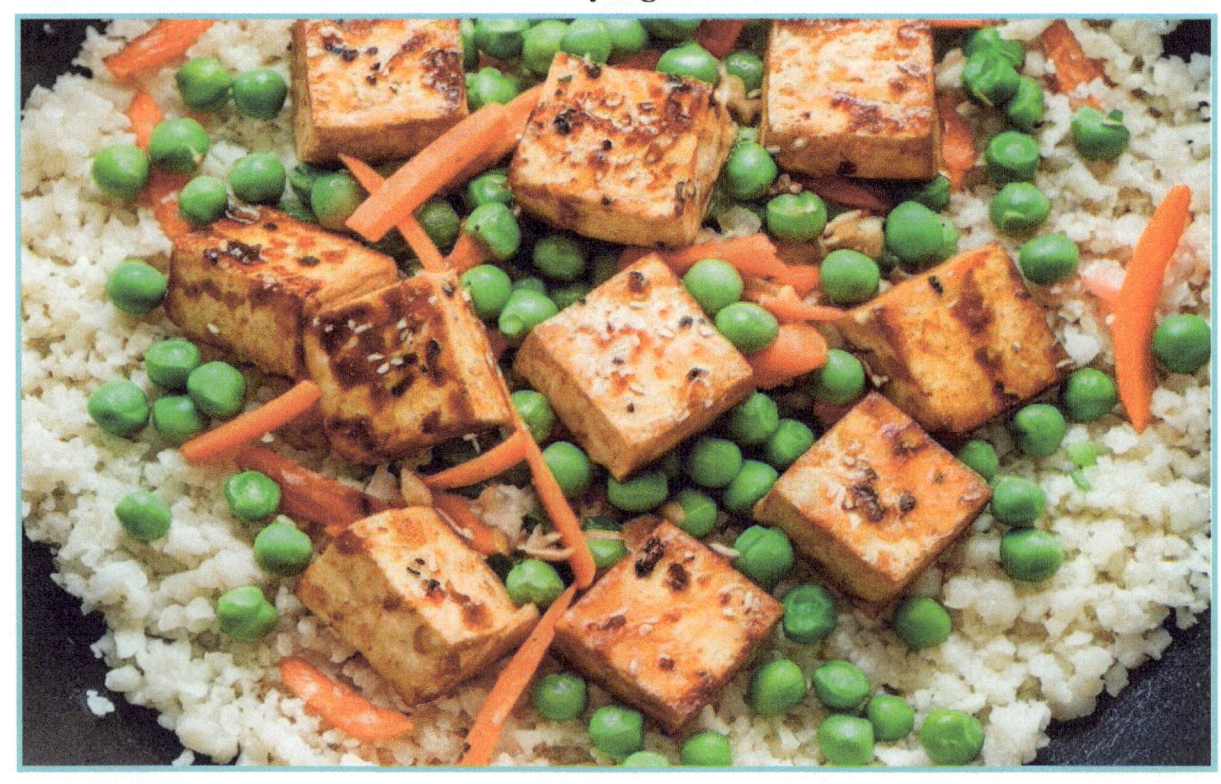

Ingredients:
- 1 cup cauliflower rice (fresh or frozen)
- 1/2 cup firm tofu, cubed
- 1/4 cup peas and carrots
- 1 tablespoon soy sauce (low-sodium)
- 1/2 teaspoon sesame oil
- 1/4 teaspoon garlic powder
- Salt and pepper, to taste

Instructions:
1. Heat sesame oil in a skillet over medium heat. Add the cubed tofu and cook for 5-7 minutes until golden and crispy on all sides.
2. Add the peas and carrots to the pan, followed by the cauliflower rice. Cook for another 5-6 minutes until the cauliflower rice is tender.
3. Stir in soy sauce, garlic powder, salt, and pepper. Serve hot.

Nutrition per Serving:
- ☐ Calories: 220
- ☐ Protein: 15g
- ☐ Fat: 12g
- ☐ Carbohydrates: 16g
- ☐ Fiber: 6g

Tip: Garnish with fresh cilantro or sesame seeds for added crunch and flavor!

Snacks: Healthy, Metabolism-Boosting

Snacking can be a great way to keep your metabolism active and maintain steady energy levels throughout the day. These healthy snacks are nutrient-dense and packed with protein, healthy fats, and fiber, which will help keep you full without spiking your blood sugar.

Recipe 1: Almond Butter and Celery Sticks

This simple yet satisfying snack is rich in healthy fats from the almond butter and fiber from the celery, making it a great option for a low-calorie day. The protein and fats will help keep you feeling full and curb cravings between meals.

Ingredients:
- 3 celery stalks, cut into sticks
- 2 tablespoons almond butter (unsweetened)

Instructions:
1. Wash and cut the celery into individual sticks.
2. Spread almond butter onto each celery stick.
3. Enjoy as a quick, satisfying snack!

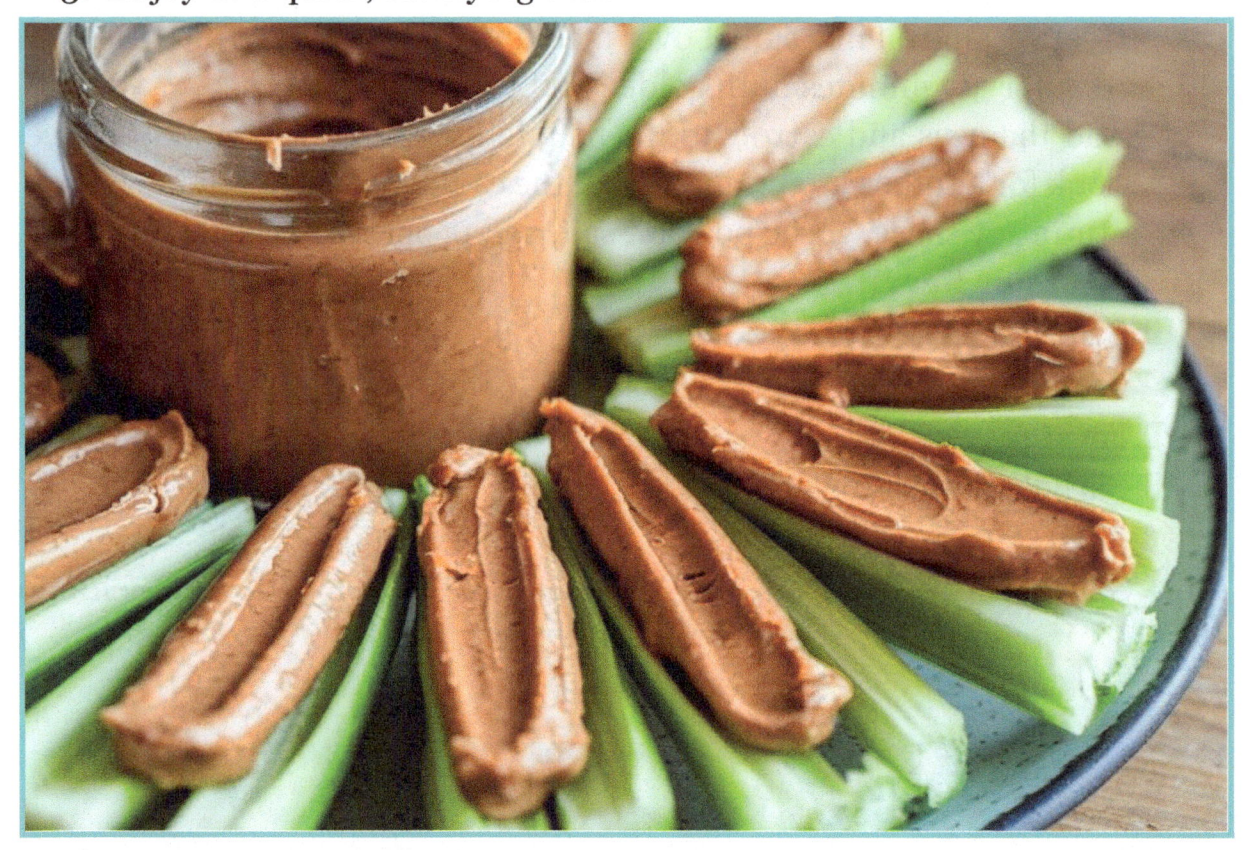

Nutrition per Serving:
- ☐ Calories: 180
- ☐ Protein: 6g
- ☐ Fat: 16g
- ☐ Carbohydrates: 7g
- ☐ Fiber: 4g

Tip: For added flavor, sprinkle a pinch of cinnamon or sea salt on the almond butter before serving.

Recipe 2: Greek Yogurt with Chia Seeds and Walnuts

This snack combines protein-packed Greek yogurt, fiber-rich chia seeds, and healthy fats from walnuts for a metabolism-boosting snack that will keep you full longer. It's perfect for a moderate-carb day or as a mid-day snack.

Ingredients:
- 1/2 cup Greek yogurt (unsweetened)
- 1 tablespoon chia seeds
- 1 tablespoon walnuts, chopped
- 1/4 teaspoon cinnamon (optional)

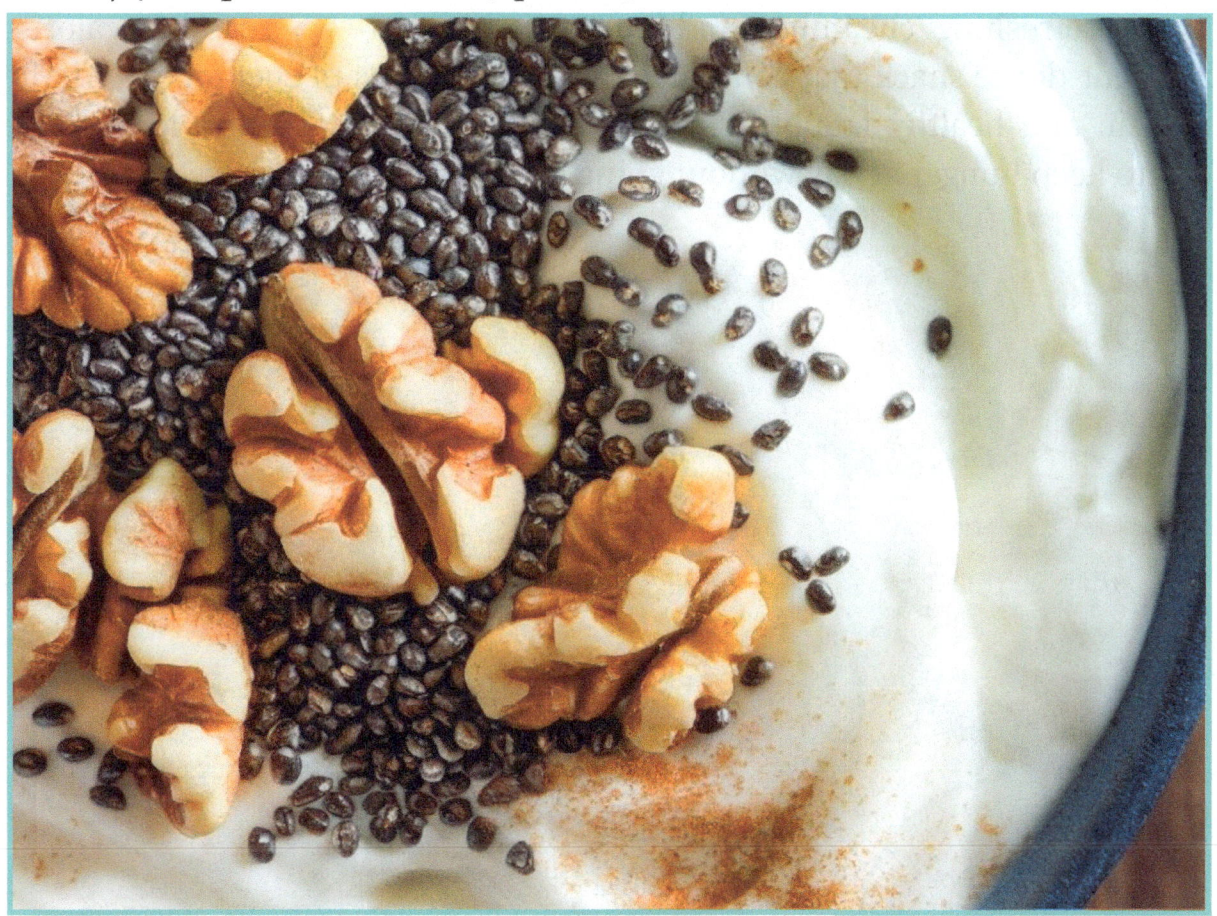

Instructions:
1. In a bowl, combine the Greek yogurt and chia seeds.
2. Top with chopped walnuts and a sprinkle of cinnamon for extra flavor.

3. Mix everything together and enjoy!

Nutrition per Serving:
- ☐ Calories: 220
- ☐ Protein: 14g
- ☐ Fat: 14g
- ☐ Carbohydrates: 12g
- ☐ Fiber: 8g

Tip: Add a few fresh berries for a natural sweetness boost and additional antioxidants.

Recipe 3: Cucumber and Hummus Bites

These refreshing cucumber and hummus bites are a great low-calorie, nutrient-dense snack that combines the cooling effect of cucumber with the protein and healthy fats of hummus. This snack is ideal for a low-calorie day to keep hunger at bay without going overboard on carbs.

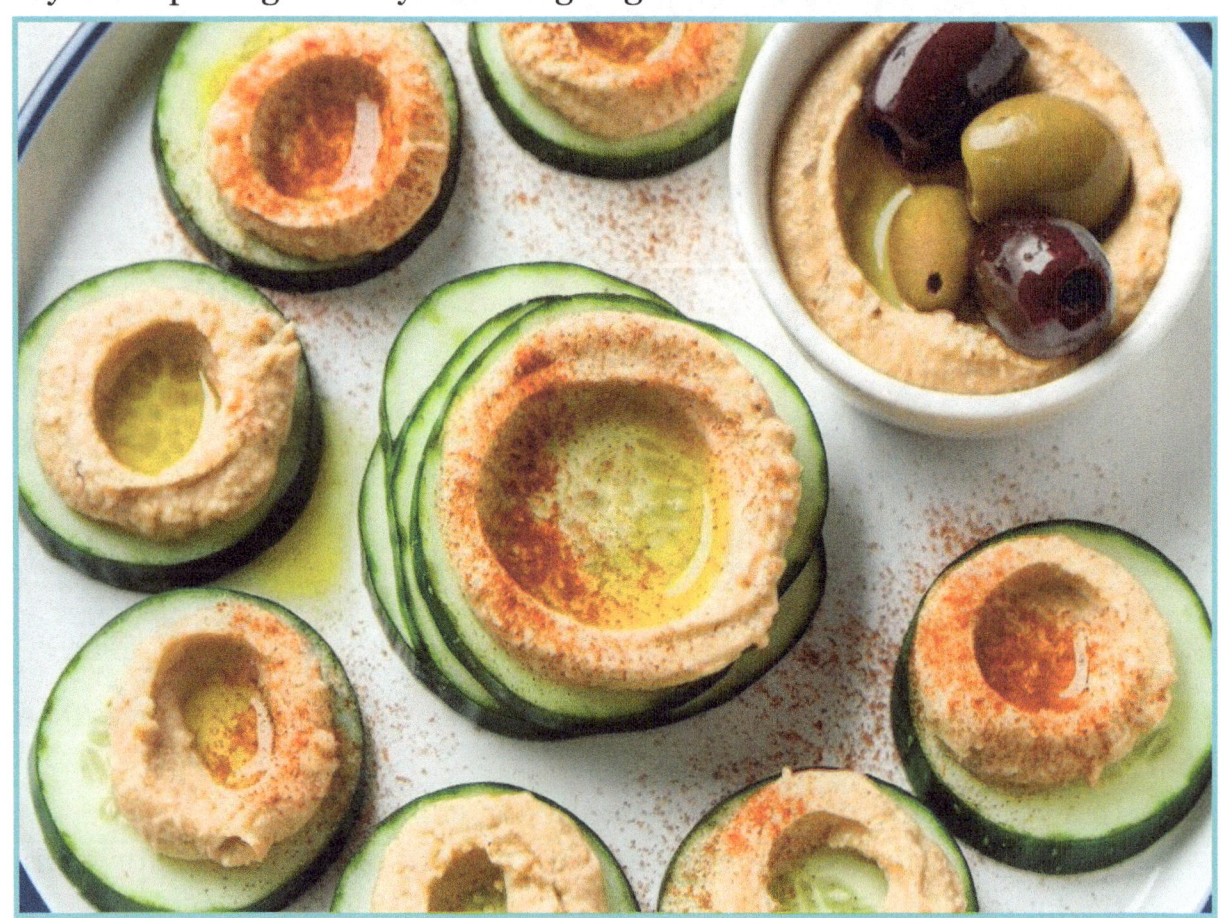

Ingredients:
- 1 cucumber, sliced into rounds
- 3 tablespoons hummus (choose a flavor you enjoy)

Instructions:
1. Slice the cucumber into thin rounds.
2. Scoop a small amount of hummus onto each cucumber slice.
3. Arrange on a plate and enjoy!

Nutrition per Serving:
- ☐ Calories: 120
- ☐ Protein: 4g
- ☐ Fat: 8g
- ☐ Carbohydrates: 10g
- ☐ Fiber: 3g

Tip: For added flavor, sprinkle with a bit of paprika or drizzle with olive oil.

Smoothies: Quick & Nutritious

Smoothies are an excellent way to pack in nutrients quickly and conveniently. These smoothies are designed to be quick, nutritious, and support your metabolism by including ingredients that help balance blood sugar, boost energy, and aid in fat loss.

Recipe 1: Green Protein Smoothie

Packed with protein, fiber, and healthy fats, this green smoothie is perfect for a moderate-carb day to keep you feeling full and energized. It's a great way to sneak in some veggies while getting a good dose of plant-based nutrition.

Ingredients:
- 1/2 cup unsweetened almond milk
- 1 scoop plant-based protein powder (or whey protein)
- 1/2 banana
- 1/2 cup spinach
- 1 tablespoon almond butter

- Ice cubes (optional)

Instructions:
1. Add almond milk, protein powder, banana, spinach, almond butter, and ice cubes to a blender.
2. Blend until smooth and creamy.
3. Pour into a glass and enjoy!

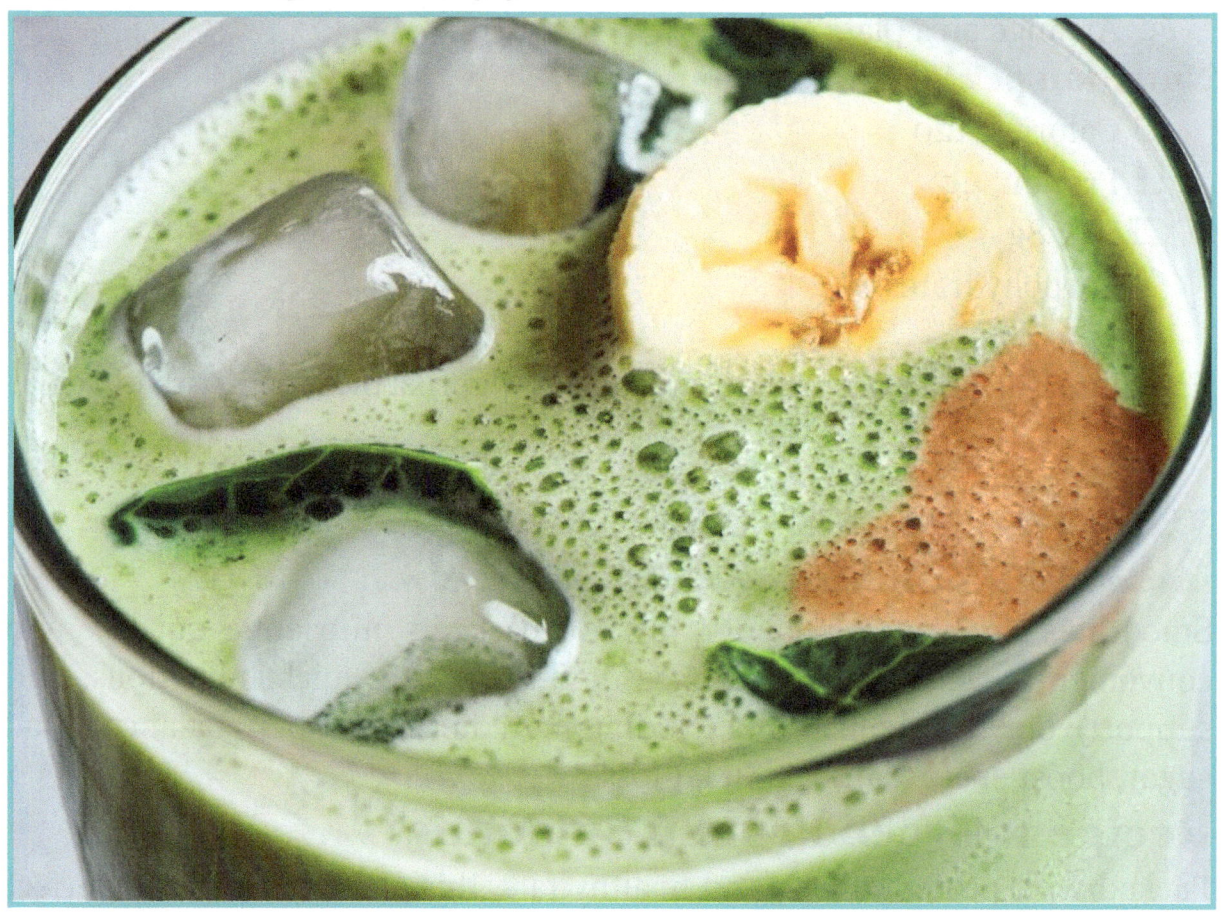

Nutrition per Serving:
- ☐ Calories: 300
- ☐ Protein: 25g
- ☐ Fat: 15g
- ☐ Carbohydrates: 18g
- ☐ Fiber: 5g

Tip: For an extra metabolism boost, add a pinch of ginger or turmeric for their anti-inflammatory properties.

Recipe 2: Berry Almond Smoothie

This berry almond smoothie is a refreshing, low-sugar option with antioxidants from the berries and healthy fats from the almonds. It's perfect for a low-calorie day when you need a quick snack that will keep you feeling full and satisfied.

Ingredients:
- 1/2 cup unsweetened almond milk
- 1/4 cup frozen mixed berries (blueberries, raspberries, or strawberries)
- 1 tablespoon almond butter
- 1 tablespoon chia seeds
- Ice cubes (optional)

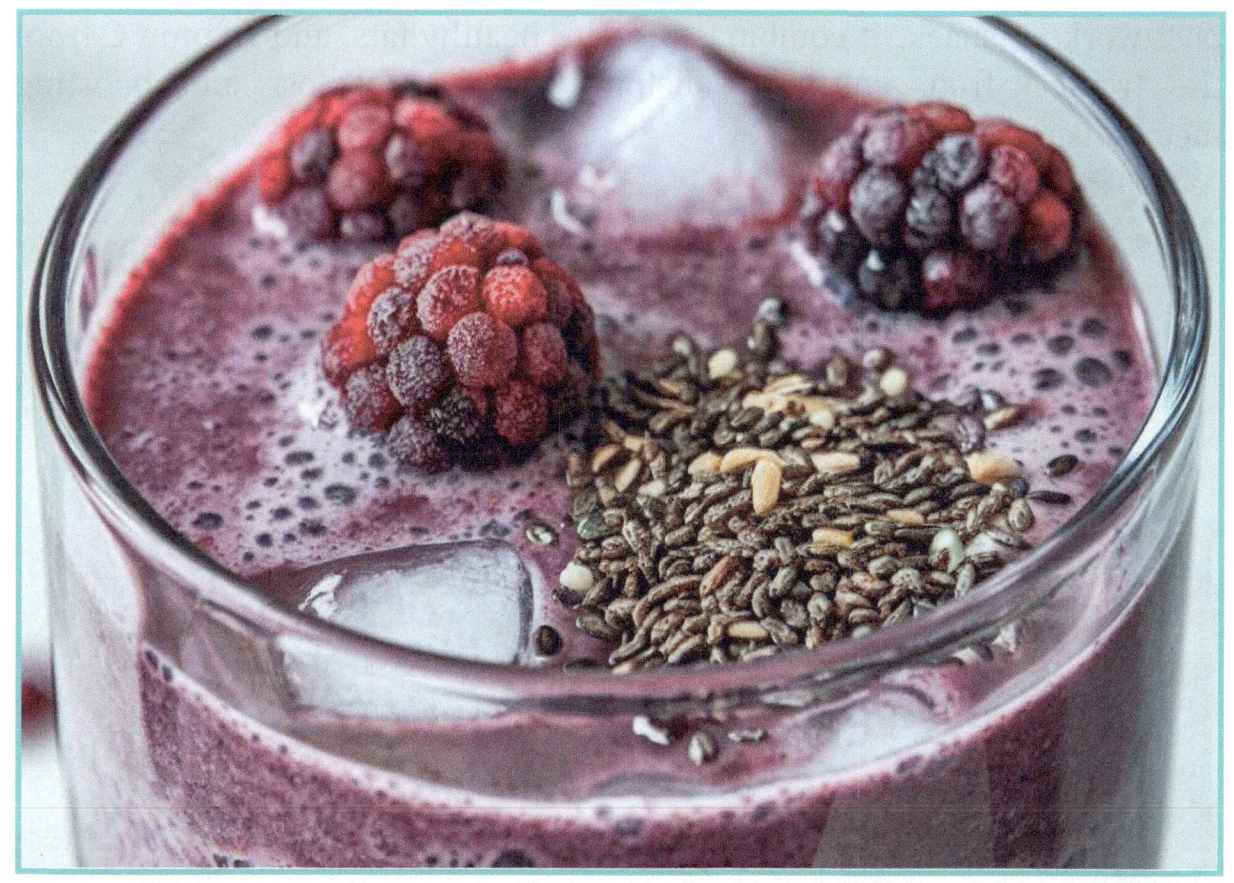

Instructions:
1. Combine almond milk, mixed berries, almond butter, and chia seeds in a blender.
2. Blend until smooth, adding ice for a thicker texture if desired.

70

3. Serve immediately.

Nutrition per Serving:
- ☐ Calories: 220
- ☐ Protein: 7g
- ☐ Fat: 14g
- ☐ Carbohydrates: 18g
- ☐ Fiber: 9g

Tip: For added protein, you can include a scoop of protein powder or Greek yogurt.

Recipe 3: Tropical Energy Smoothie

This tropical smoothie is perfect for a quick, nutrient-packed breakfast or post-workout snack. It combines protein, healthy fats, and vitamin C from the tropical fruits, all while helping support fat loss and boosting metabolism.

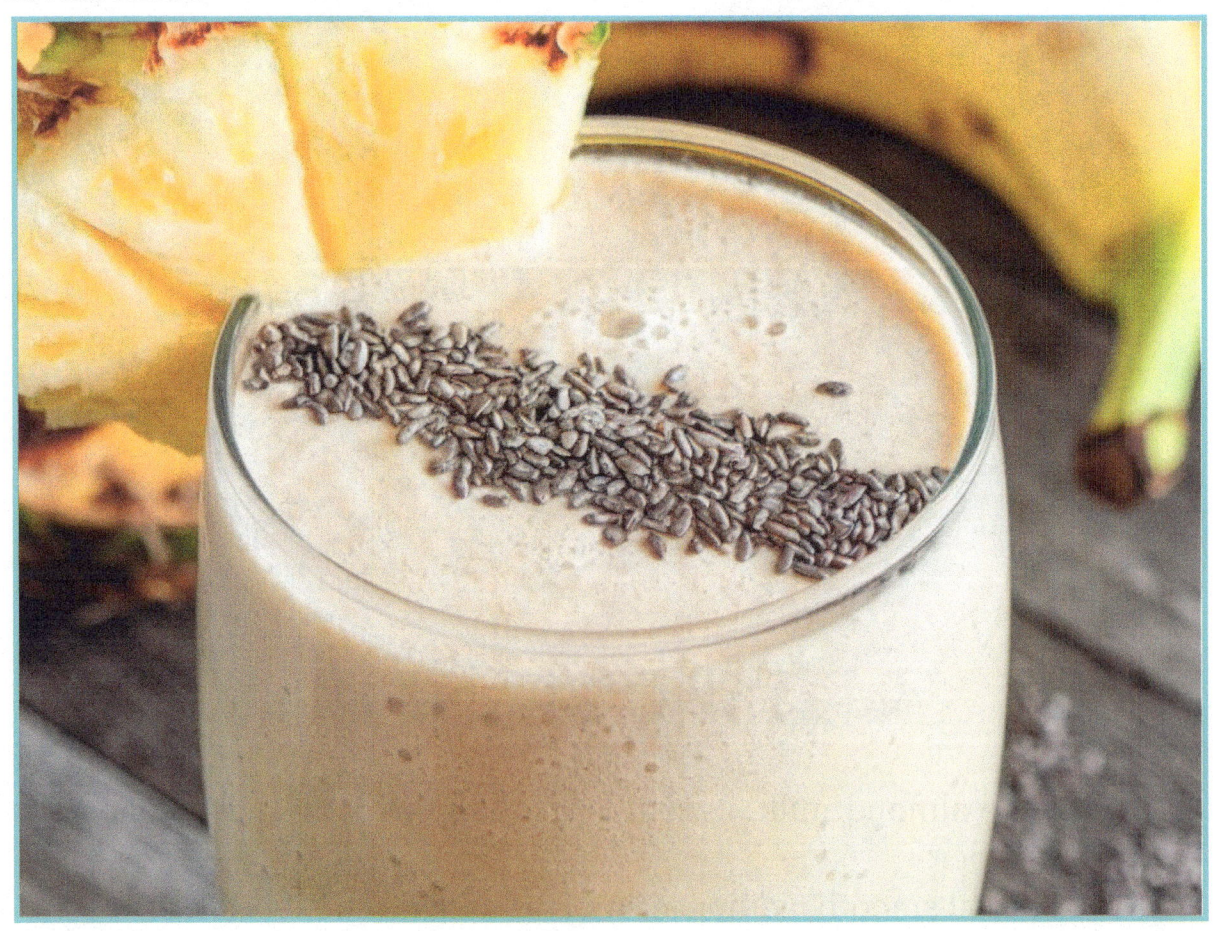

Ingredients:
- 1/2 cup unsweetened coconut milk
- 1/2 cup frozen pineapple chunks
- 1/2 banana
- 1 tablespoon coconut oil
- 1 scoop collagen protein powder (optional)
- Ice cubes (optional)

Instructions:
1. Add coconut milk, pineapple, banana, coconut oil, and collagen protein to a blender.
2. Blend until smooth and creamy, adding ice if you prefer a colder smoothie.
3. Pour into a glass and enjoy!

Nutrition per Serving:
- Calories: 280
- Protein: 12g
- Fat: 20g
- Carbohydrates: 22g
- Fiber: 4g

Tip: You can add a handful of spinach for extra nutrients without altering the taste much.

Desserts: Sweet and Supportive

Who says you can't enjoy a little sweetness while sticking to your Metabolic Confusion Diet? These sweet and supportive desserts are designed to satisfy your cravings without derailing your progress. Packed with healthy ingredients and metabolism-boosting benefits, these desserts are perfect for anyone who wants to indulge while staying on track.

Recipe 1: Chocolate Avocado Mousse

This rich and creamy mousse is made with avocado, which adds healthy fats and a silky texture, while the cocoa powder gives it a delicious chocolatey flavor. It's a perfect dessert for a low-calorie day, providing healthy fats without the sugar crash.

Ingredients:
- 1 ripe avocado, peeled and pitted
- 2 tablespoons unsweetened cocoa powder
- 2 tablespoons almond milk (or any milk of choice)
- 1 tablespoon honey or maple syrup (optional, for sweetness)
- 1/2 teaspoon vanilla extract
- Pinch of salt

Instructions:
1. Place all ingredients in a blender or food processor.
2. Blend until smooth and creamy. If the mousse is too thick, add a little more almond milk to reach the desired consistency.
3. Taste and adjust sweetness, adding more honey or maple syrup if desired.
4. Chill in the refrigerator for at least 30 minutes before serving.
5. Serve with a sprinkle of cocoa nibs or chopped almonds for crunch.

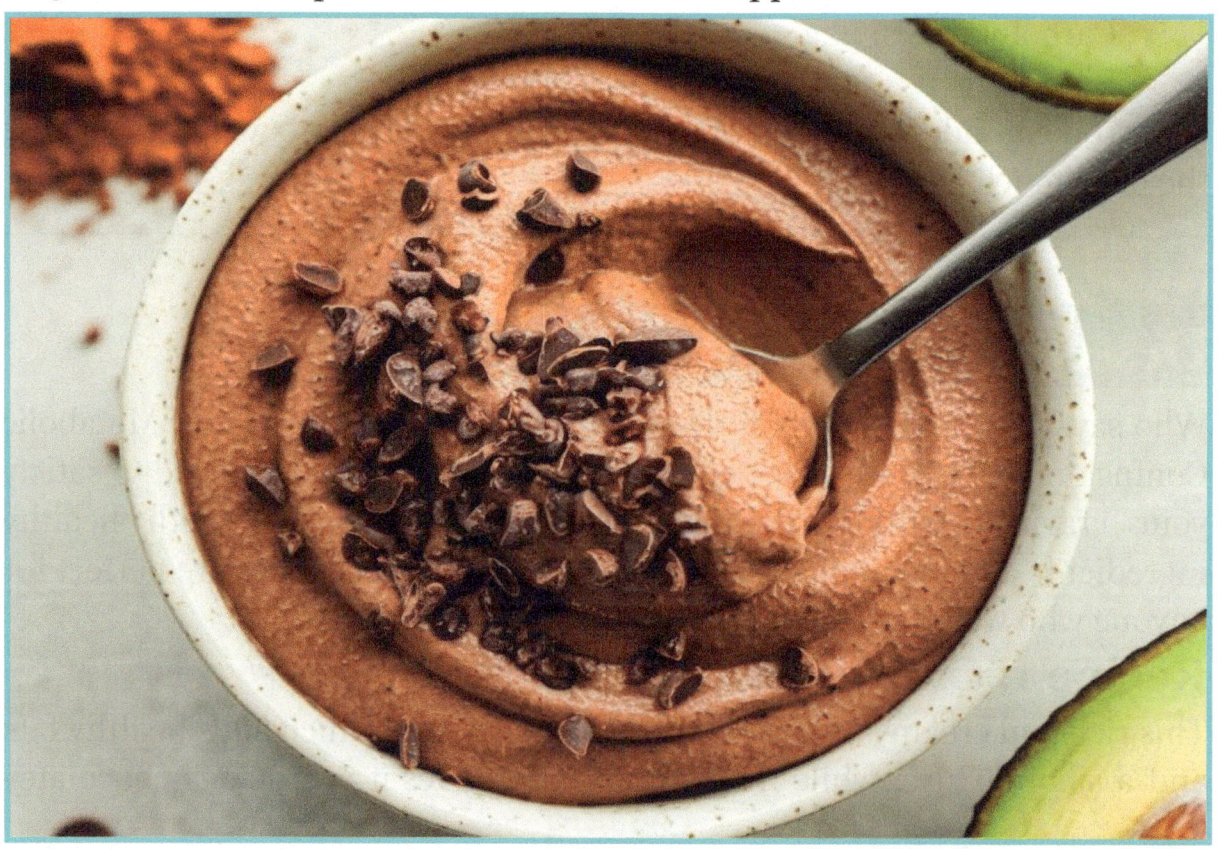

Nutrition per Serving:
- Calories: 220
- Protein: 3g
- Fat: 18g
- Carbohydrates: 16g
- Fiber: 9g

Tip: This mousse can be made ahead of time for an easy, healthy dessert option during the week.

Recipe 2: Coconut Chia Pudding

This chia pudding combines coconut milk and chia seeds to create a rich, creamy dessert that's packed with healthy fats and fiber. It's perfect for a moderate-carb day, offering a satisfying, sweet treat without compromising your goals.

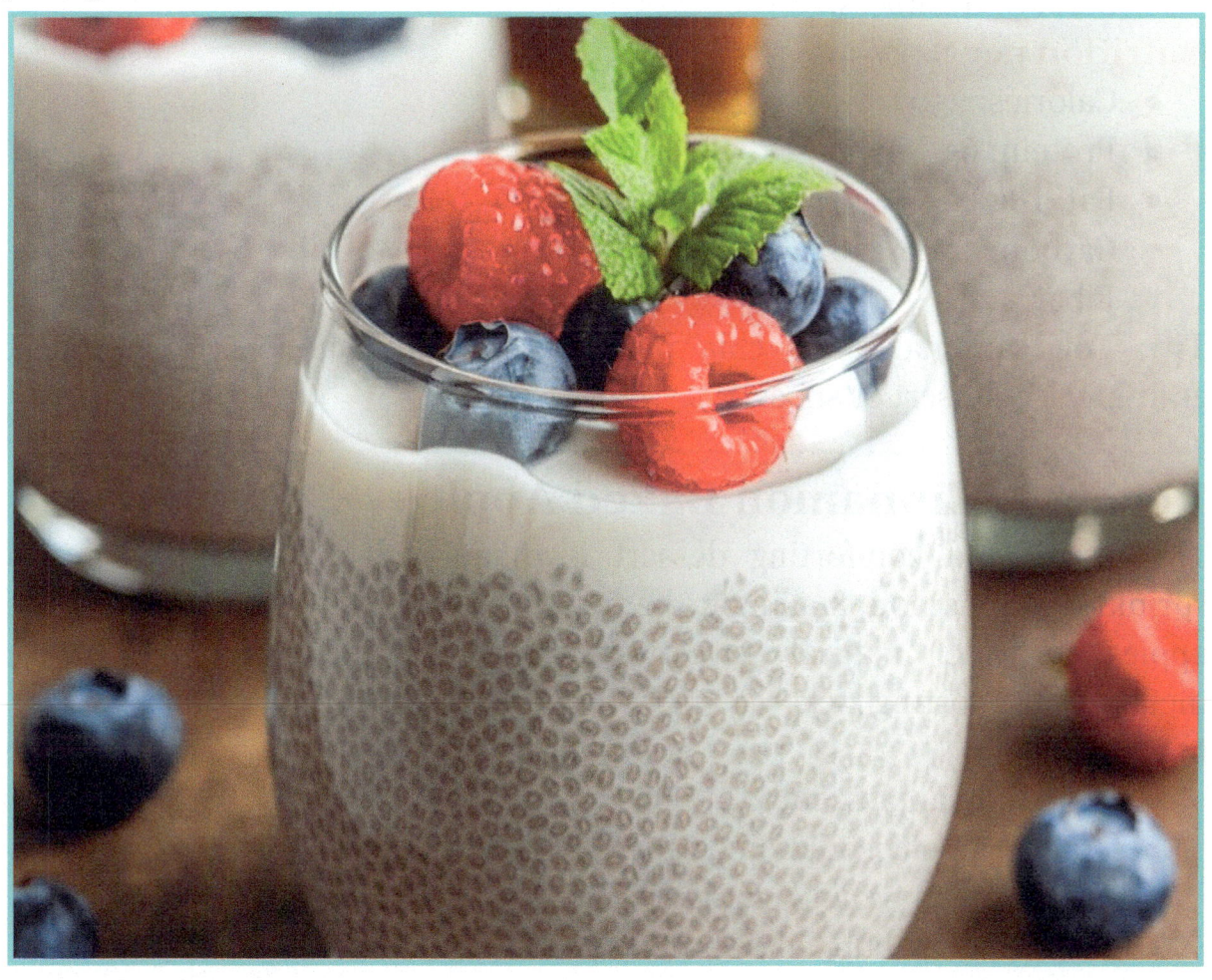

Ingredients:
- 1/2 cup canned coconut milk (unsweetened)
- 1/2 cup unsweetened almond milk
- 3 tablespoons chia seeds
- 1 tablespoon maple syrup or honey (optional)
- 1/4 teaspoon vanilla extract
- Fresh berries (for topping)

Instructions:
1. In a bowl or jar, combine the coconut milk, almond milk, chia seeds, maple syrup, and vanilla extract.
2. Stir well to combine, ensuring the chia seeds are evenly distributed.
3. Cover and refrigerate for at least 4 hours or overnight to allow the chia seeds to absorb the liquid and thicken.
4. Top with fresh berries before serving for added antioxidants and a burst of freshness.

Nutrition per Serving:
- Calories: 250
- Protein: 6g
- Fat: 18g
- Carbohydrates: 18g
- Fiber: 12g

Tip: You can make this chia pudding in individual jars for a quick, grab-and-go dessert or snack!

Recipe 3: Cinnamon Baked Apples

This warm and comforting dessert is made with baked apples and a sprinkle of cinnamon, making it the perfect treat for a low-calorie day. The apples provide natural sweetness, and the cinnamon adds a metabolism-boosting kick.

Ingredients:
- 2 medium apples, cored
- 1 tablespoon coconut oil (melted)
- 1/2 teaspoon ground cinnamon
- 1 tablespoon chopped walnuts (optional)

- 1 tablespoon almond butter (optional)

Instructions:
1. Preheat the oven to 375°F (190°C).
2. Core the apples, creating a hollow space in the center.
3. Place the apples in a baking dish and drizzle with melted coconut oil. Sprinkle cinnamon on top.
4. Optional: Stuff the apples with chopped walnuts for added crunch or a small dollop of almond butter for extra richness.
5. Bake for 20-25 minutes, or until the apples are tender.
6. Serve warm, and enjoy!

Nutrition per Serving:
- Calories: 180
- Protein: 3g
- Fat: 10g
- Carbohydrates: 22g
- Fiber: 6g

Tip: Serve with a dollop of Greek yogurt for extra protein and a creamy texture.

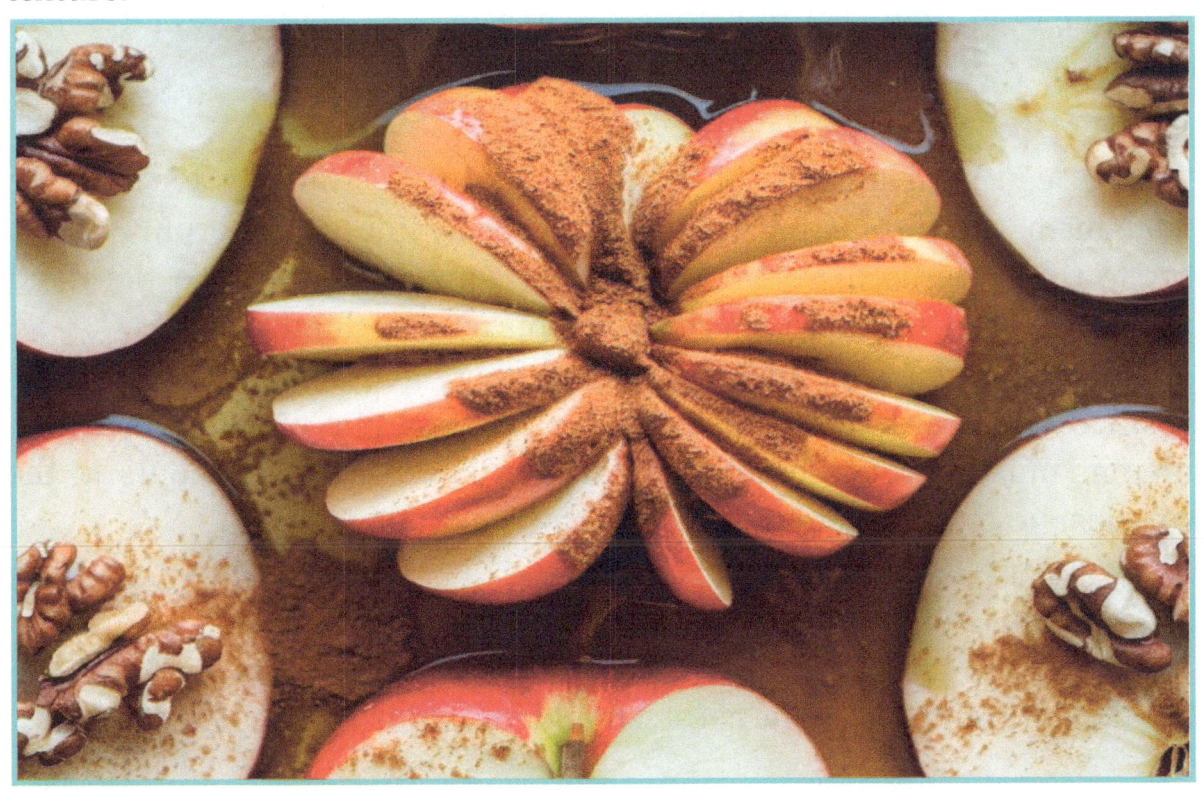

Part V: Exercise & Lifestyle

When it comes to Metabolic Confusion and achieving your weight loss and energy goals, combining the right nutrition with the best exercise routine is crucial. For endomorph women, who tend to have a slower metabolism and may struggle with fat loss, focusing on the right types of exercise can make a huge difference. The goal is to build lean muscle, boost metabolism, and promote fat burning. Let's dive into the best workouts for endomorph women to maximize results!

Best Workouts for Endomorph Women

For endomorph women, the key to an effective workout routine is balance. You'll want to focus on a combination of strength training, cardio, and high-intensity interval training (HIIT). These workouts not only help build lean muscle, which boosts metabolism, but also burn fat efficiently. Below are the best types of workouts that will work in harmony with your Metabolic Confusion Diet to help you achieve your weight loss and fitness goals.

1. Strength Training (3-4 Days a Week)

Building lean muscle is one of the most important strategies for boosting metabolism and promoting fat loss, especially for endomorph women. Muscle tissue burns more calories at rest compared to fat, so the more muscle you build, the more calories you'll burn throughout the day.
—Strength training can include weightlifting, bodyweight exercises, or resistance band workouts. Aim for 3-4 sessions per week, focusing on different muscle groups each day. You don't need to spend hours in the gym—just 30 to 45 minutes per session can make a big impact.

Key Strength Training Moves:
- Squats: Great for targeting the legs and glutes.
- Deadlifts: Target the lower back, glutes, and hamstrings.
- Push-ups: Focus on the chest, shoulders, and triceps.

- Rows (with dumbbells or resistance bands): Strengthen the back and biceps.
- Lunges: Work the legs and glutes while improving balance.

Tip: Focus on compound movements (like squats, deadlifts, and lunges) that engage multiple muscle groups at once. These exercises are more effective for fat loss and muscle building.

2. High-Intensity Interval Training (HIIT)

HIIT is one of the most effective workouts for fat burning, especially for endomorph women who may have a harder time losing fat. HIIT involves short bursts of intense exercise followed by a brief rest period. It's perfect for keeping your metabolism revved up long after the workout is over.

—HIIT can be done with various exercises, including bodyweight movements or using equipment like kettlebells, dumbbells, or a treadmill. The idea is to push yourself during the intense periods to elevate your heart rate and burn fat while maintaining muscle mass.

Sample HIIT Workout for Endomorph Women:
- ☐ 30 seconds of jumping jacks
- ☐ 30 seconds of rest
- ☐ 30 seconds of squat jumps
- ☐ 30 seconds of rest
- ☐ 30 seconds of push-ups
- ☐ 30 seconds of rest
- ☐ 30 seconds of mountain climbers
- ☐ 30 seconds of rest

Repeat this circuit 3-4 times for a full workout.

Tip: HIIT workouts can be completed in just 20-30 minutes, making them an excellent option if you're short on time. They are incredibly efficient for burning fat while preserving muscle.

3. Cardiovascular Exercise (2-3 Days a Week)

Cardio workouts are essential for burning calories and supporting heart health, but for endomorph women, it's important to find a balance. While excessive cardio can potentially lead to muscle loss, moderate cardio is great for fat loss and boosting your metabolism.

—Aim for 2-3 cardio sessions per week, and mix up the intensity and duration. This could include brisk walking, jogging, cycling, swimming, or using machines like the elliptical or rowing machine. For fat burning, try a combination of steady-state cardio (like a moderate-intensity walk or jog) and higher-intensity sessions, depending on how your body responds.

Types of Cardio:
- Moderate-intensity cardio: Brisk walking, light jogging, or cycling for 30-45 minutes.
- Interval cardio: Alternating between higher-intensity bursts (like sprinting) and lower-intensity recovery periods.

Tip: Use cardio as a supplement to your strength training and HIIT routine. Focus on quality over quantity when it comes to cardio—moderate amounts are enough to enhance fat loss and improve cardiovascular health.

---

4. Active Recovery (1-2 Days a Week)

While strength training, HIIT, and cardio are important, don't overlook the benefits of active recovery. Endomorph women can sometimes overtrain without realizing it, which can lead to burnout or even injury. Active recovery focuses on activities that help your body recover without stressing it further.

Active recovery could include activities like:
- **Yoga**: Helps with flexibility, stress relief, and muscle recovery.
- **Walking**: A gentle way to keep the body moving without overloading it.
- **Stretching**: Improves mobility and can help with recovery after intense workouts.

Tip: Active recovery is just as important as the more intense workouts. It helps your muscles repair and grow while keeping you active and motivated.

---

5. Consistency and Progression

The best results come from consistent and progressive training. While mixing up your workouts is important to prevent plateaus, it's equally essential to keep increasing the intensity of your workouts over time. This could be through:
- Increasing the weight you lift.
- Adding more repetitions or sets.
- Increasing the duration or intensity of your cardio.
- Trying more advanced versions of exercises as you progress.

Tip: Track your workouts and aim for gradual improvements. Even small increases in intensity or effort will have a big impact over time!

Lifestyle Tips: Sleep, Stress, Hydration

1. Sleep: The Foundation of Recovery

Getting enough quality sleep is one of the most important factors in weight loss, muscle recovery, and overall health. Sleep directly affects your metabolism, hunger hormones, and energy levels, which are crucial for sticking to your Metabolic Confusion Diet and workout plan.

Why Sleep Matters:
- Regulates Hormones: Lack of sleep can disrupt key hormones like ghrelin (hunger hormone) and leptin (satiety hormone), leading to increased cravings and overeating.
- Boosts Metabolism: Sleep plays a key role in fat metabolism and muscle recovery. A rested body is more efficient at burning fat and building muscle.
- Reduces Stress: When you're well-rested, you're better equipped to handle daily stressors, preventing emotional eating or poor food choices.

Sleep Tips:
- Aim for 7-9 hours of quality sleep each night.
- Establish a sleep routine by going to bed and waking up at the same time each day (even on weekends).
- Keep your sleep environment dark, cool, and quiet for the best rest.

- Limit screen time (phones, computers, TVs) at least 30-60 minutes before bed to help your body relax.

2. Stress: Managing Stress for Better Results

Stress can interfere with weight loss by increasing cortisol levels, which promote fat storage, especially around the belly. Managing stress is essential for maintaining a healthy metabolism and avoiding emotional eating.

Why Stress Matters:
- Increases Cortisol: High levels of cortisol, the stress hormone, can cause your body to hold onto fat, particularly in the abdominal area.
- Affects Sleep: Chronic stress can lead to poor sleep quality, which, as mentioned, negatively impacts metabolism and hunger regulation.
- Leads to Emotional Eating: Stress often triggers emotional eating or cravings for comfort foods, which can sabotage your progress.

Stress Management Tips:
- Practice deep breathing exercises or try meditation for 5-10 minutes each day to help reduce stress levels.
- Try incorporating yoga or gentle stretching into your routine to calm the mind and body.
- Engage in hobbies or activities you enjoy to take your mind off stress (reading, gardening, painting, etc.).
- Take breaks throughout the day to reset and avoid burnout, especially if you're feeling overwhelmed.

3. Hydration: Keeping Your Body Fueled and Energized

Drinking enough water is critical for optimal metabolism, fat loss, and muscle function. Staying hydrated also helps with digestion, energy levels, and curbing hunger, making it easier to stick to your calorie cycling and meal plan.

Why Hydration Matters:
- Boosts Metabolism: Dehydration can cause your metabolism to slow down, making it harder to burn fat efficiently.

- Reduces Hunger: Sometimes, thirst is confused with hunger. Drinking water can help control unnecessary cravings and prevent overeating.
- Improves Exercise Performance: Staying hydrated ensures your muscles are functioning properly during workouts, improving endurance and strength.

Hydration Tips:
- Aim to drink at least 8 cups (64 ounces) of water a day. More may be needed if you're physically active or live in a hot climate.
- Start your day with a glass of water to kickstart hydration.
- Drink water before meals to help curb hunger and promote digestion.
- If you find plain water boring, try adding lemon, mint, or cucumber for flavor.

Tracking Progress & Staying Motivated

Tracking your progress and staying motivated are key to maintaining long-term success with your Metabolic Confusion Diet. Weight loss and fitness are journeys, and consistency is what drives results. Here's how you can track your progress and stay motivated throughout the process.

1. Tracking Progress: Celebrate Your Wins

Tracking progress isn't just about the number on the scale—it's about recognizing all the small victories along the way. By tracking your progress, you can identify what's working, what needs tweaking, and celebrate your successes.

How to Track Progress:
- Track Your Weight and Body Measurements: While the scale is a tool, it's important to track other indicators of progress, like waist circumference, hip measurements, and body fat percentage. These measurements often reveal fat loss that the scale might not show.

- Take Progress Photos: Sometimes, visual changes are more apparent than numbers. Take a full-body photo every 2-4 weeks to compare and see the differences.
- Track Your Workouts: Keep a workout journal to track the intensity, reps, and sets of your strength training and HIIT sessions. Progress in strength and stamina means your metabolism is working!
- Monitor Energy and Sleep: Pay attention to how your energy levels and sleep patterns improve as you stick to your diet and exercise routine.

Tip: It's important to track non-scale victories such as feeling stronger, fitting into clothes better, or simply having more energy to get through the day. These are all signs of progress!

2. Staying Motivated: Keep Your Eyes on the Prize

Staying motivated over the long haul can be tough, but with the right strategies, it's easier to keep your momentum going.

Motivation Tips:
- Set Specific, Achievable Goals: Break your larger weight loss and fitness goals into smaller, manageable milestones. For example, aim to lose 1-2 pounds per week or increase your squat weight by 5-10 pounds over the next month.
- Find a Workout Buddy: Having a workout partner can help you stay accountable and make exercise more enjoyable.
- Mix Up Your Routine: Variety is key to preventing burnout. Change up your workout routine every few weeks to keep things fresh and exciting.
- Reward Yourself: Set up a reward system where you celebrate small victories. Treat yourself to something special (like a massage or new workout gear) after reaching a milestone.

Tip: When motivation wanes, remind yourself of why you started. Whether it's for improved health, confidence, or energy, reconnecting with your "**why**" can reignite your passion.

Part VI: Troubleshooting

As you follow the Metabolic Confusion Diet, you may encounter a few bumps along the way. Whether it's a weight loss plateau, unexpected life changes, or common mistakes that hinder your progress, it's important to have strategies in place to overcome these challenges. This section will help you troubleshoot any roadblocks and stay on track toward your goals.

Overcoming Plateaus

Plateaus are a common part of any weight loss journey, and they can be frustrating. However, a plateau doesn't mean you've failed—it simply means your body has adapted to your routine and needs a little adjustment to keep progressing. Here are some strategies to help you break through a weight loss plateau:

1. Reevaluate Your Calorie Intake

Your body may have adapted to your calorie cycling pattern, which could slow down your progress. If you've been following the same routine for a while, try slightly adjusting your calories. For example, you might need to increase your calories on high-calorie days or reduce them on low-calorie days.

- Increase your high-calorie days by adding an extra serving of protein or healthy fats.
- Reduce your low-calorie days slightly to create a bigger calorie deficit.

2. Change Your Workout Routine

Your body can get used to the same workouts, which can lead to a plateau in fat loss and muscle growth. Changing up your routine can help reactivate your metabolism and continue progressing.

- Increase the intensity of your workouts (e.g., adding more weight to your strength training or increasing your HIIT intervals).
- Try different exercises to target muscles in new ways and avoid adaptation. For example, if you've been doing bodyweight squats, try adding dumbbells or kettlebells.

- Add more cardio (moderate-intensity or HIIT) if you feel your body can handle it without overtraining.

3. Focus on Non-Scale Victories

Sometimes, the scale doesn't reflect the progress your body is making. Focus on other signs of success like:
- Increased strength or stamina in your workouts.
- Better sleep quality and increased energy levels.
- Clothing fitting better, even if the scale isn't budging.

This will help you stay motivated and keep moving forward, even when the scale is stuck.

4. Check Your Stress and Sleep Levels

High stress and poor sleep can contribute to plateaus by affecting hormones like cortisol, which can promote fat storage. Make sure you're managing stress and getting adequate sleep to support your weight loss and overall well-being.

Adjusting for Life Changes

Life is unpredictable, and changes in your schedule, environment, or health can sometimes throw a wrench in your progress. Whether it's a change in your work routine, travel, or a busy family life, it's important to adjust your Metabolic Confusion Diet to maintain consistency without feeling overwhelmed.

1. Adjust Your Meal Prep Routine

If you're busy or traveling, you can still stick to your Metabolic Confusion meal plan with a little preparation:
- Batch cook your meals for the week in advance, so you have healthy options ready to grab when life gets hectic.
- If you're traveling, look for hotel room-friendly meals (e.g., salads with lean protein, snack bars with protein, or ready-made meals that align with your diet).

2. Incorporate Flexible Exercise

If your schedule gets busy and you can't hit the gym as often, try to fit in shorter, more efficient workouts at home. Even a 10-minute HIIT session or a quick bodyweight workout can help maintain your metabolism and prevent a setback.

- Morning or lunchtime workouts can help you stay consistent on busy days.
- Take the stairs or go for a brisk walk if you can't find time for a full workout.

3. Manage Stress During Life Changes

Life transitions (e.g., starting a new job, moving, or family stress) can raise cortisol levels, which can lead to weight gain or difficulty losing fat. Implement strategies like mindfulness, yoga, or simple breathing exercises to help manage stress and keep your cortisol levels in check.

4. Adapt to Health Changes

If you experience an injury or other health concerns, focus on adjusting your workouts accordingly. Low-impact exercises like swimming, cycling, or yoga can still support your metabolism and fat loss without stressing your body.

Common Mistakes & Solutions

While following the Metabolic Confusion Diet, it's easy to make a few common mistakes that can slow progress. Here are some of the most frequent pitfalls and how to avoid them:

1. Not Tracking Calories or Macronutrients Accurately

Sometimes, even if you're following a plan, small errors in calorie or macronutrient tracking can prevent weight loss. Be sure you're measuring your food properly and tracking everything that goes into your mouth, even snacks and condiments.

Solution:
- Use a food scale to measure portions accurately.

- Track your food using an app or journal to ensure you're staying within your calorie and macronutrient goals.

2. Skipping High-Calorie Days

Some people think that eating fewer calories every day will lead to faster weight loss, but this can actually hinder your metabolism. Skipping high-calorie days can cause your body to slow down its fat-burning process.

Solution:

- Stick to your calorie cycling plan—don't skip your high-calorie days, as they're important for keeping your metabolism active and preventing fat storage.

3. Overdoing Cardio

While cardio is important for fat loss, doing too much can lead to muscle loss and slow down your metabolism, especially for endomorph women who already have a slower metabolism. Excessive cardio can also lead to burnout and fatigue, making it harder to stick with your diet and exercise plan.

Solution:

- Limit your cardio sessions to 2-3 days a week, focusing on moderate to high-intensity intervals. Balance cardio with strength training to preserve muscle mass and maintain a high metabolism.

4. Not Getting Enough Protein

Protein is essential for building muscle and maintaining a strong metabolism. If you're not getting enough protein, your body might burn muscle instead of fat, which can slow down your metabolism and hinder fat loss.

Solution:

- Make sure to include lean protein in every meal and snack (e.g., chicken, turkey, fish, tofu, or legumes) to support muscle growth and repair.
- Aim for about 1.2 to 1.6 grams of protein per kilogram of body weight per day.

5. Focusing Only on the Scale

It's easy to get discouraged if the scale isn't moving, but weight isn't the only indicator of success. Your body composition (muscle mass versus fat mass), how your clothes fit, and your energy levels matter just as much.

Solution:
- Focus on non-scale victories like improved strength, better sleep, more energy, or feeling more confident.
- Take progress photos and measurements to track changes in your body composition over time.

In Summary:
- Plateaus are a normal part of the process, but they can be overcome by adjusting your calorie intake, changing up your workout routine, and focusing on non-scale victories.
- Life changes (work, family, health) may require adjustments to your meal prep, exercise routine, and stress management strategies to stay on track.
- Common mistakes include inaccurate tracking, skipping high-calorie days, overdoing cardio, and neglecting protein intake. Avoiding these mistakes and staying consistent with your routine will help you stay on course.

The key to overcoming obstacles is adaptation. Stay flexible, track your progress, and make adjustments when needed. By incorporating these troubleshooting strategies, you'll continue progressing toward your goals and maintain long-term success with your Metabolic Confusion Diet.

Conclusion

Congratulations on taking the first step toward achieving your health, fitness, and weight loss goals with the Metabolic Confusion Diet! By now, you've learned how to harness the power of calorie cycling, build a tailored meal plan, incorporate the best exercises for your body type, and implement key lifestyle habits like sleep, stress management, and hydration. This holistic approach not only supports fat loss but also promotes muscle building, boosts energy, and enhances overall well-being.

—But remember, this journey is not just about hitting a specific number on the scale—it's about transforming your body, feeling more confident, and taking control of your health. Success comes from consistency, patience, and making small adjustments along the way. You'll encounter challenges, and that's okay! The important thing is to stay committed, listen to your body, and continue progressing at your own pace.

Here's a recap of key takeaways:

- Metabolic Confusion helps keep your metabolism active, prevents plateaus, and optimizes fat loss by alternating between high- and low-calorie days.
- Focus on strength training, HIIT, and moderate cardio to boost metabolism, burn fat, and build lean muscle.
- Support your efforts with lifestyle habits like getting enough sleep, managing stress, and staying hydrated.
- Track your progress through measurements, photos, and how you feel—don't just rely on the scale.
- Adapt as life changes and stay consistent with your diet and workouts to maintain long-term success.

As you continue on this path, remember that each small step you take is moving you closer to your ultimate goal. Celebrate your victories, stay motivated, and trust the process.

—You've got this! Here's to unlocking a healthier, stronger, and more energized you. Keep going, stay consistent, and enjoy the journey. You're capable of achieving amazing results—and this is just the beginning!

Bonus Content

Welcome to the bonus section of your Metabolic Confusion Diet journey! In this section, you'll find helpful resources that will make sticking to your meal plan even easier, such as a grocery list for beginners, meal prep tips, and printable meal plan templates to help you stay organized and on track. Let's dive in!

Grocery List for Beginners

A well-stocked kitchen is essential to staying on track with your Metabolic Confusion Diet. Here's a beginner-friendly grocery list that includes everything you need for your first few weeks. This list is designed to provide you with healthy, whole foods that will support your calorie cycling and meal planning.

Protein Sources:
- ☐ Chicken breast (skinless)
- ☐ Ground turkey (lean)
- ☐ Salmon or other fatty fish (like mackerel or sardines)
- ☐ Eggs (organic, if possible)
- ☐ Tofu (for plant-based options)
- ☐ Greek yogurt (unsweetened)
- ☐ Canned beans (black beans, chickpeas)
- ☐ Cottage cheese (unsweetened)

Healthy Fats:
- ☐ Avocados
- ☐ Almond butter or peanut butter (unsweetened)
- ☐ Olive oil (extra virgin)
- ☐ Coconut oil
- ☐ Chia seeds
- ☐ Walnuts, almonds, or other nuts
- ☐ Flaxseeds (optional, for smoothies)

Vegetables:
- ☐ Spinach (fresh or frozen)
- ☐ Kale (fresh or frozen)
- ☐ Broccoli (fresh or frozen)
- ☐ Zucchini
- ☐ Cauliflower
- ☐ Bell peppers
- ☐ Asparagus
- ☐ Cucumbers
- ☐ Tomatoes (cherry or regular)
- ☐ Carrots (baby or regular)
- ☐ Mixed greens (for salads)
- ☐ Sweet potatoes (for moderate-carb days)

Fruits:
- ☐ Berries (blueberries, raspberries, strawberries)
- ☐ Apples
- ☐ Bananas (for smoothies or snacks)
- ☐ Lemons (for dressings and flavor)
- ☐ Pineapple (fresh or frozen)

Whole Grains & Carbs:
- ☐ Quinoa
- ☐ Brown rice
- ☐ Oats (for breakfast or snacks)
- ☐ Whole wheat bread or wraps (optional, for higher-calorie days)
- ☐ Sweet potatoes (for moderate-carb days)
- ☐ Dairy (Optional):
- ☐ Unsweetened almond milk (or any plant-based milk)
- ☐ Unsweetened coconut milk (for cooking or smoothies)
- ☐ Cheese (like feta or goat cheese, optional for salads)

Herbs & Spices:
- ☐ Fresh parsley or cilantro

- ☐ Garlic (fresh or powder)
- ☐ Onion powder
- ☐ Ground turmeric
- ☐ Cinnamon
- ☐ Smoked paprika
- ☐ Salt and pepper
- ☐ Miscellaneous:
- ☐ Tahini (for dressings)
- ☐ Soy sauce (low-sodium)
- ☐ Balsamic vinegar
- ☐ Mustard (for dressings or marinade)
- ☐ Protein powder (whey or plant-based, if desired)
- ☐ Coconut flakes (unsweetened, optional for smoothies or desserts)

Meal Prep Tips

Meal prepping is one of the best ways to stay on track with your Metabolic Confusion Diet. It saves time during the week and ensures that healthy meals are always available. Here are some meal prep tips to make it easier:

1. Plan Your Meals Ahead of Time

Spend some time each week planning out your meals for the next 3-4 days. Write down your breakfast, lunch, dinner, and snacks so you know exactly what to buy and prepare.

Use printable meal plan templates (included below) to organize your week's meals and ensure you're getting the right balance of protein, carbs, and fats for your calorie cycling days.

2. Batch Cook and Portion

Cook in large batches. Prepare proteins (chicken, turkey, salmon), vegetables (broccoli, zucchini, cauliflower), and carbs (quinoa, sweet potatoes, brown rice) at the beginning of the week.

Portion out meals into individual containers. This will make it easier to grab a pre-made meal during busy days, and it ensures that you stick to your portion sizes.

3. Use Freezer-Friendly Containers

If you're not able to eat everything in a few days, store meals in freezer-safe containers. Freezing portions ensures they last longer and will save you time during the week.

When reheating, use a microwave or stove for best results—avoid using the oven to retain the moisture in the food.

4. Pre-Chop Veggies and Prep Snacks

Pre-chop veggies for salads, snacks, or stir-fries. This makes it easier to throw together a meal without much effort.

Pre-portion snacks like almond butter with celery sticks or Greek yogurt with chia seeds so they're ready to grab.

5. Keep It Simple and Stick to Your Staples

Choose simple, easy-to-make recipes that you can repeat throughout the week. Dishes like salads, stir-fries, and protein bowls are great options.

Stick to your grocery list of staple ingredients, and try to rotate between them for variety. For example, rotate between chicken breast, turkey, and tofu for protein, or sweet potatoes, quinoa, and brown rice for carbs.

Printable Meal Plan Templates

To help you stay organized and on track with your Metabolic Confusion Diet, here are some printable meal plan templates that you can download and use each week. These templates will help you visualize your meals, track your calorie cycling pattern, and ensure you're eating a balanced diet.

Weekly Meal Plan Template

- **Breakfast**: Plan your high-protein, low-carb or moderate-carb breakfasts for each day.
- **Lunch**: Include a variety of protein, healthy fat, and vegetable combinations. Don't forget to incorporate different carb options (for moderate-carb days).

- **Dinner**: Plan low-calorie or balanced meals, depending on your goals. Include lean proteins and vegetables.
- **Snacks**: Keep your snacks balanced with protein and healthy fats. Include things like Greek yogurt, nuts, and veggies with hummus.

You can create your own weekly plan or use a pre-filled template based on your specific needs.

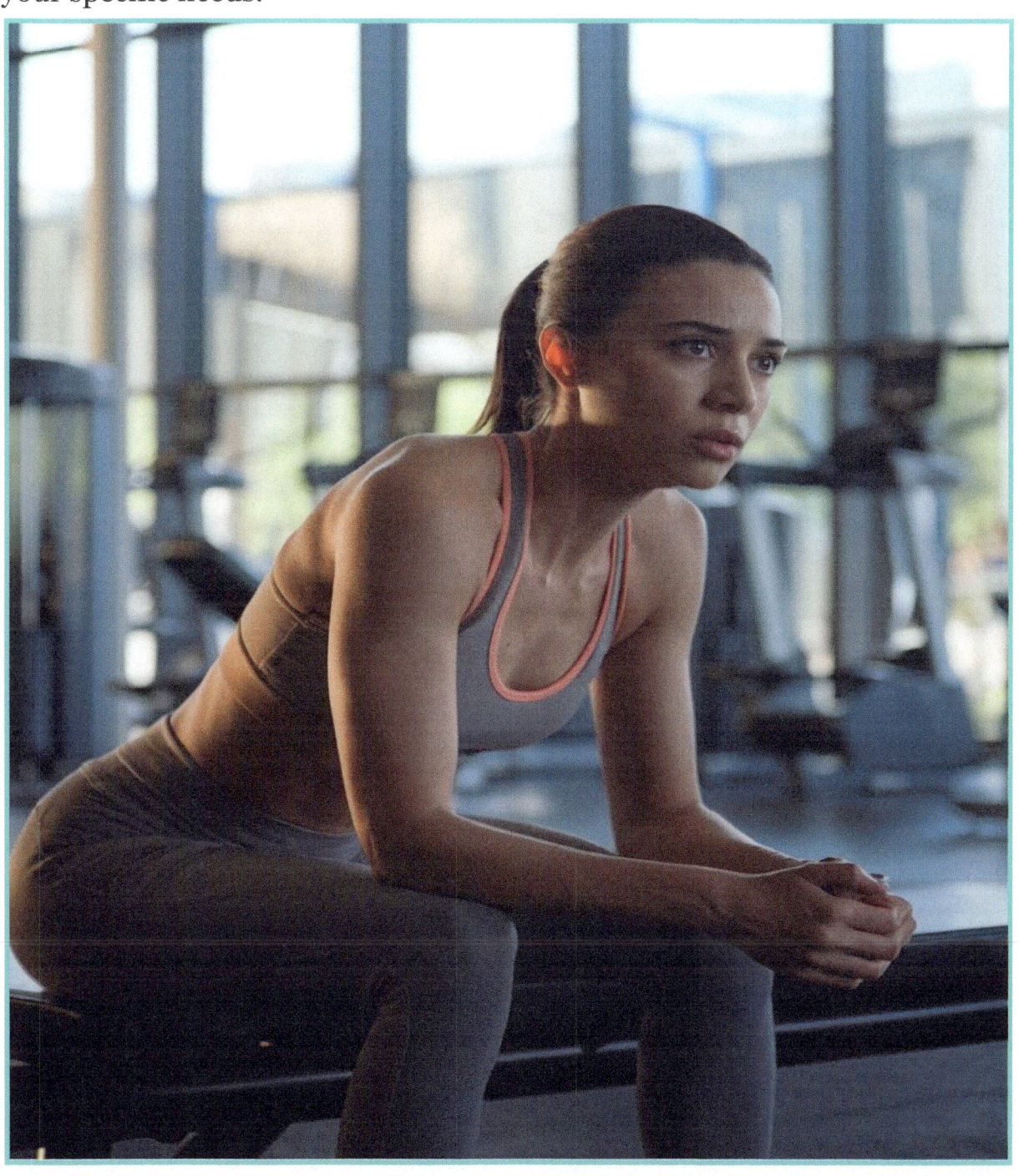

Made in the USA
Las Vegas, NV
04 April 2025